Staying Power

Staying Power

Maintaining Your Low-Carb Weight Loss for Good

Michael R. Eades, M.D.

Mary Dan Eades, M.D.

WILEY

John Wiley & Sons, Inc.

Published by John Wiley & Sons, Inc., Hoboken, New Jersey
Published simultaneously in Canada

Design and composition by Navta Associates, Inc.

For general information about our other products and services, please contact our Customer Care Department within the United States at (800) 762-2974, outside the United States at (317) 572-3993 or fax (317) 572-4002.

Wiley also publishes its books in a variety of electronic formats. Some content that appears in print may not be available in electronic books. For more information about Wiley products, visit our web site at www.wiley.com.

Library of Congress Cataloging-in-Publication Data:

Eades, Michael R.
   Staying power : maintaining your low-carb weight loss for good /
Michael R. Eades and Mary Dan Eades.
      p. cm.
  Includes index.
  ISBN-10 0-471-72566-8 (cloth)
  ISBN-13 978-471-72566-4 (cloth)
 1. Low-carbohydrate diet. I. Eades, Mary Dan. II. Title.
  RM237.73.E233 2005
  613.2'83—dc22

                               2005001250

Printed in the United States of America

10 9 8 7 6 5 4 3 2 1

Dedicated to our granddaughter,
Emma Alexandra Rockefeller Eades,
the first girl in the Eades line in a long time

Contents

Acknowledgments ix

Introduction 1

CHAPTER 1 Are You Ready for Maintenance? 5

CHAPTER 2 Transition: The Journey Begins 11

CHAPTER 3 Maintenance: One Size Fits You 35

CHAPTER 4 Maintenance: The Balancing Act 49

CHAPTER 5 Answers to All Your Low-Carb Questions 73

APPENDIX A Protein Requirements 130

APPENDIX B Protein and Carbohydrate Servings Lists 132

APPENDIX C Meal Planner Worksheet 144

APPENDIX D The Staying Power LifePlanner 145

Index 255

Acknowledgments

No book is a singular work, certainly not this one. We owe a debt of gratitude to all the people who helped make this project a reality.

First, as always, our thanks go to our faithful agents, Carol Mann and Channa Taub, for their tireless efforts on our behalf.

Many thanks to our editor, Tom Miller, and all the fine people at John Wiley & Sons who worked day and night to get this book between the covers and onto the shelves in record time.

We gratefully acknowledge the help of our sister/sister-in-law, Rose Crane, for her efforts in compiling quotes and tips, and to our nurse, Debbie Nelson Judd, for her work compiling questions and answers from readers and patients; both were integral to the creation of this book. And to our never-tiring assistant, Kristi McAfee, thanks for all you do keep the empire humming along while we work.

Our gratitude also goes to all our patients and corresponding readers over the years, who have taught us much about how to help people do the hard work of weight maintenance.

And last, but certainly not least, to our family—our wonderful sons, Ted, Dan, and Scott, our beautiful daughters-in-law, Jamye and Katherine, and our grandangels, Thomas, Will, and Emma. All we do, we do for you.

Introduction

This book is not a diet book per se. It's not about weight loss or lowering your cholesterol or blood sugar. Rather, *Staying Power* is a guidebook to help you learn how to hang onto the health and weight goals you've worked so hard to achieve. It's about maintenance—the end game. If you've lost weight on a low-carb diet, this may become one of the most important books in your dietary library.

Without a doubt, what follows "the diet" is the most difficult, but arguably the most important, phase of any nutritional plan. And yet, in the past, the maintenance phase of dieting has received precious little ink; it was usually tossed off as a coda to a weight-loss plan. Sure, most diet books (including all of our previous works) address the topic of maintenance, but too often in a lip-service chapter at the end of a long book on how to lose the weight, drop cholesterol, or control blood pressure. The pro forma bows to maintenance usually run something like this: now that you're thinner and healthier, it's important to stay that way, and if you eat like you've been eating, you will. You know what to do; just do it! Period.

In fact, if your life stayed on an even keel and you continued to eat the way you were eating when you lost weight and regained your health, maintenance probably would be a snap. All the millions of people who lose billions of pounds every year would join the ranks of the lean and healthy, and soon obesity, diabetes, and heart disease would be things of

the past. We'd be the leanest nation on earth, not the fattest. But the
hard truth is that weight maintenance eludes ninety-five out of one
hundred successful dieters. By far and away, most people who lose
weight on any kind of diet—including rigorous fasting regimens or even
stomach-stapling procedures—will regain most of it within a year. Sadly,
many of them will regain all they lost and more. And with the regain will
come the return of all the health issues that the healthful weight loss
solved. Sounds pretty bleak, and it is, but with the right guidance, it
needn't be. Maintenance will be a challenge. It will require effort and
some measure of sacrifice, but it's far from impossible. It can be done,
and you can do it!

During our twenty years of helping people lose weight and solve
their weight-related health problems, we confronted the bogeyman that
is maintenance right from the beginning with all of our patients. We told
them that losing weight is the easy part, maintaining it the crucial part.
Maintenance really is the name of the game. A weight-loss diet is just a
tool to get you to the point where you can begin the real work of making
the lifestyle changes stick. Weight loss should never be viewed as an end
in itself; rather, it's the beginning of a new life in maintenance.

If you've successfully lost weight and solved your weight-related
issues on a low-carb diet, whether by following the recommendations of
one of our books (*The 30-Day Low-Carb Diet Solution*, *Protein Power*, or
The Protein Power LifePlan) or by going on Atkins or the Zone, heading
to South Beach, or using any of the many low-carb plans that have burst
upon the scene, your challenge now is learning to live in sync with this
dietary philosophy over the long haul. Trust us when we say that if low
carb got you thin and well, then, as our Southern grandmothers used to
say, you need to "dance with him that brung you" and learn to maintain
that way. If you responded favorably to the low-carb regimen, if you lost
weight, lowered your cholesterol and triglycerides, and controlled your
blood sugar or blood pressure, you've proven beyond a shadow of a
doubt that you have a tendency toward insulin resistance and some or all
of the disorders that it can cause. Controlling carbs to some extent will be
the lynchpin of your maintenance success. Do not kid yourself that it
could be otherwise. As we told our patients again and again, if we could
bop you on the head with a magic wand and "Poof!" make you instantly
lean and healthy, you wouldn't stay that way for long if you didn't make a

sea change in the way you eat and live. Accepting and internalizing this truth is the first great challenge of your maintenance. If you try to go back to your old way of eating, we'll make you a guarantee right here and now: you'll go back to your old weight and state of health.

But maintenance is more than just a way of eating. It's a way of life, a way of thinking about what's important to you, and a way of prioritizing which things are important enough to make long-term changes, even sacrifices, for. Because maintenance isn't a destination; it's a journey. And on the way, you'll encounter smooth sailing and tough going. You'll hit snags and enjoy successes. To tackle the work of maintenance, you need a road map to help you sidestep the pitfalls and anticipate the turbulence that may threaten to unhinge your commitment. You'll also need a game plan in place to repair short-term damage when it occurs and to get you quickly back on track. *Staying Power* will provide these important tools.

We have constructed a careful stepwise maintenance plan like the one we used successfully for nearly twenty years with our patients. It will guide you week by week as you make the transition from weight loss and health correction and begin your maintenance journey. We'll share stories from our patient files illustrating common pitfalls that can undermine your maintenance success, and we'll provide coping strategies that lessen their impact. We've devised delicious meal plans for breakfasts, lunches, dinners, and even snacks to guide you nutritionally along the way, as you gradually liberalize your carb intake and allow your body to ease its way into a new balance. When life throws you a curve, our strategies for flexibility will keep you in the game and will restore your balance.

But the centerpiece of this maintenance game plan is the 365-day Staying Power LifePlanner journal you'll use to record your progress. In our experience, there's no better way to cement your new lifestyle than by keeping a careful record for a substantial period of time. Your daily journal is a handy place to record the carbohydrate content of all your meals and snacks and the amount and the type of exercise you do, as well as your fluid and dietary supplement intake. Every week, you'll find helpful nutritional tips and uplifting quotes to motivate you, along with space to chart your vital statistics and set forth goals. We cannot overemphasize the importance of keeping a careful journal to ensure your long-term success. When you make a life change, whether it's quitting smoking, sticking to an exercise plan, or improving your diet, research has shown that you'll be *four times more likely to succeed* if you put it all in writing than if you don't. *Staying Power* provides an easy way for you to keep track of the information that you need to make your low-carb maintenance plan work for years to come.

We've designed the journal in a universal format, not specific to a particular year, so that no matter when you start on the path to maintenance, you'll have 365 days—a full calendar year—to solidify your new maintenance lifestyle. Again, we, didn't just randomly choose the year-long format; clinical research has proved that people who maintain their weight correction for a full year are far more likely to succeed in keeping the weight off for the long haul than those who do not.

A year in maintenance will see you through every important date on your calendar—all the family birthdays, your anniversary, summer vacation, as well as the traditional secular and religious feasting holidays that can so easily undermine your commitment to staying on course. A year in maintenance will give you an opportunity to pinpoint almost all the potential dietary trouble spots in your life: eating on the run or on the road, business lunches Monday through Friday, traditional ballpark food every Friday night from August through December, Aunt Betty's coconut cream pie on Sundays after church, the ice cream parlor between the office and the bus stop after work, and the holiday food frenzy that starts with "Trick or treat!" and ends with "Happy New Year!"

Every maintenance journey is different; what appeals to one person might not cause even a flicker of temptation in someone else. Your goal is to figure out what works for *you*. Use your journal every day to discover where your own temptation traps lie and to develop a workable counter-strategy to sidestep them, and you'll be well on your way to a lifetime of health and weight maintenance.

CHAPTER 1

Are You Ready for Maintenance?

In general, two categories of dieters can answer yes to that question: those who have reached or are nearing their final goals in weight or health parameters and those who have reached an interim goal and want to take a break from corrective diet mode for a time. Both groups will find great help here. In general, because the low-carb diet is so effective at solving weight-related health issues, the decision to set an interim goal usually involves weight loss, rather than health. For most people, serious low-carb dieting effectively corrals the health issues wrought by an unruly metabolism in a matter of a few months, but even at 2 to 4 pounds per week, it takes time to accomplish significant weight loss.

We'd like to speak first to dieters who have reached an interim goal and ask you to examine why you're taking a diet break and whether doing so is the right course for you. Although there may be any number of good reasons for taking a break before you've achieved your goal, be aware that some people find it more difficult to get back into the weight-loss mind-set after relinquishing it. Based on our years of clinical experience, we honestly think that the best course of action, when feasible, is to buckle down and push on through the corrective phase to your goal and then maintain. In this matter, you really must know yourself. If staying with the modest rigors of corrective low-carb dieting will levy a burden either physically or emotionally at this time, that's reason enough to take a breather and maintain for a while. If you've lost your diet mind-set, are stuck on a plateau, and seem to be struggling in vain to progress, it's a good time to examine the reasons why you may be stuck and what to do about them. You'll find answers that address overcoming plateaus in chapter 5, "Answers to All Your Low-Carb Questions." It may also help you to think of the corrective phase, however long it may take, as a diet boot camp, sometimes demanding, sometimes requiring sacrifice, not always pleasant, but in the end very good for you.

The obvious exception to this general advice would be during pregnancy. Quite often, we've noticed, young women experience reproductive hormonal alterations during weight loss and, surprise! They discover that they've become pregnant. Pregnancy is an obligatory reason to take a break from losing weight. Under no circumstances should a pregnant woman undertake a reduced-calorie weight-loss diet. On the other hand, a healthy carb-controlled maintenance diet is quite good for pregnant women. It has plenty of fresh fruits and veggies; protein from meats, eggs, and poultry; good quality fats; dairy products; and some whole grains and is limited in sugar and refined starches. It's an obstetric dietitian's dream diet.

How, you may ask, do you know when you're near enough to your goals to begin maintenance? Here are some guidelines:

- If you set weight loss as a goal when you began your low-carb diet, you should now be within 10 pounds of your ideal body weight. (If you had very little weight to lose at the outset, you should be within 3 to 5 pounds of your goal.) It's important to realize that you will likely continue to lose a few more pounds in the first weeks of maintenance.

- If you were working to correct health issues, your cholesterol, triglycerides, blood pressure, or blood sugar should have returned to near-normal levels.

- Bad heartburn or gastroesophageal (GE) reflux should be a dim and distant memory.

- You should be sleeping soundly and waking more rested, with greater energy than before.

Now is the time to take a Progress Chart to measure your current status against where you were when you started a low-carb plan. You'll find the worksheets in the back of the book.

Take stock now, by measuring and weighing yourself, assessing your clothing sizes, and repeating any abnormal blood tests that were health issues when you began the program. See how far you've come toward the goals you first set for yourself. If, after doing so, you still feel that you've got more work to do in correcting your weight or health issues, continue (or return to) corrective dieting for a bit longer.

If, on the other hand, you've nearly accomplished what you set out to do, then you've made it to the end of corrective dieting and are ready to begin the transition into maintenance for a lifetime of good health in a leaner body.

Elizabeth's Story: Don't Be Afraid to Maintain

Most people, after spending several months or more restricting their carb intake to 7 to 10 grams per meal, look forward with great anticipation to the luxury of graduating to a higher carbohydrate intake. Most, but certainly not all, relish taking the next step. Occasionally, though, in our practice, we've encountered some resistance. Our patient Elizabeth comes to mind.

Elizabeth came to us in her early 30s, about 45 pounds overweight but otherwise relatively healthy. She embraced the corrective phase of her low-carb diet with great vigor, even creating some delicious recipes that she shared with other patients. Thanks to her commitment and focus, she made steady, strong progress toward her goal weight, week after week. In less than six months, she was within striking distance of it. When she came into the clinic for her transition visit, we were excited to see her take this next step on her journey toward maintenance. Yet she seemed somewhat subdued—not her usual upbeat self. We discussed her progress, with which she was clearly delighted, and then outlined our recommended changes in diet therapy to ease her carbohydrate intake upward.

The following week when she returned to the clinic, her diet journal showed that she still hadn't added any additional carbohydrates. She had continued to eat at the corrective level—in fact, eating almost exactly the same meals as the week before. Nothing much had changed, except that she'd lost about half a pound more weight. Our dietitian repeated the new game plan, and Elizabeth assured her that she would comply, but at her next visit a week later, she was still eating at the corrective level.

When our nursing staff asked why, Elizabeth replied that she was terrified to advance. The corrective diet had been so easy and effective, and she was so pleased with the way she looked and felt that she didn't want to rock the boat. She strongly believed that indulging in too many high-carb foods had caused her weight to climb in the first place. In this, she was correct; she'd developed a real weakness for donuts and pastries, during and after her pregnancy several years earlier, and rightly felt that adherence to the low-carb diet had been instrumental in her being able to kick the habit. She hadn't so much as tasted a donut in months and finally didn't miss them. And now, she feared that relinquishing her restraint on carbs even slightly might open the floodgates of carb craving and sweep away her success.

This feeling of apprehension is not that uncommon in people who have struggled with their weight and finally gained control. And it's quite true that returning to old habits, to the unrestrained eating of excessive empty, concentrated carbs will indeed pave the road to weight regain. But eating reasonable quantities of healthy, nutrition-packed carbs will not.

It took some convincing, but we gradually persuaded Elizabeth to increase her carbs slightly, with larger, but still just moderate-sized, servings of low-starch vegetables and fruits. We assured her that in the unlikely event this small increase might cause her weight to inch upward, she could always drop back to the corrective carb level and stay there indefinitely without any compromise to her long-term health. She could simply bump up her calories from protein and good-quality fats sufficiently to stop her weight loss and maintain at the 7- to 10-grams-per-meal level of carbs. You see, the rationale for increasing carb content is not health concerns. As long as you focus on quality in your carb selection, even 40 to 50 grams of effective carbs a day in fresh fruits and vegetables (such as green leafies, tomatoes, peppers, squashes, green and cruciferous vegetables, lower-carb root veggies, such as celery root and jicama, along with berries, melons, and lower-sugar fruits) will provide more than enough alkalinity to protect your bones. The rationale is to afford your palate more variety and a broader spectrum of naturally occurring antioxidant compounds, micronutrients, and other phytochemicals and to make the maintenance diet so delicious and inclusive that you'll easily be able to stick to it for life.

We promised Elizabeth that our game plan wouldn't fail her, and we'll make that promise to you as well. If you have any qualms about being able to increase your carb intake and maintain your weight, don't fret. Just take it slowly and easily, and make every added carb count nutritionally. Recognize that there will be a carb limit for everyone, some higher than others. If at any time in the course of increasing your daily carb intake, you find that you gain weight or your clothing seems tight for no apparent reason, simply return to the corrective level, drop the extra pound or two, hang out there a while, and (as our toddler grandsons would say) try and try again.

The Softer Benefits of Living Life in Maintenance

What you have already accomplished could add many years of good health and happiness to your life! Take a moment to give yourself some well-deserved kudos and to think about the many benefits that losing weight and gaining control of your health have brought you. Based on what thousands of patients and readers have told us in the past, we're sure you're enjoying life in ways you may never have imagined. Perhaps you are now taking part in activities with your family and friends that you once avoided because of poor health, fatigue, or overweight. Perhaps you can now keep up with your children or grandchildren without becoming out of breath or exhausted. Maybe, as so many of our patients and readers have done, you've taken up a new active hobby. Some of our patients have become involved in everything from competitive country-western line dancing and power lifting to kickboxing, kung fu, marathon running, surfing, and hang gliding. Reclaiming your health and fitness will reinvigorate your life. So, get out there and have fun! You've certainly earned it. And it's only going to get better.

Maybe you now enjoy being able to shop for clothes anywhere you want, buying what's fashionable instead of having to settle for what fits, buying a new pair of jeans that feels—and looks—good. Often the small changes have the greatest positive impact on your life: being able to cross your legs comfortably when you sit, no longer feeling compelled to suck in your stomach all day long, forsaking stretch pants forever. And sometimes, things that seem inconsequential to one person are of huge psychological and emotional importance to another: not having to request a seatbelt extender on the airplane, being light enough for your son to pick you up and twirl you around, being able to weigh yourself again on a regular bathroom scale, or not being chosen last for softball. All of these benefits were experienced and related to us by our patients and readers.

We'd be remiss not to mention the other obvious benefits—the health ones. If you're like many (if not most) people who've lost weight on a low-carb diet, keeping control in maintenance means no longer having to remember to take a bevy of medications to control your blood sugar, blood pressure, cholesterol, or triglycerides—and no longer suffering from the side effects they can cause. It means not scrounging in your purse or your pocket for antacid tablets after every meal. It means that instead of spending half a car payment at the drugstore each month, you've learned to control those disorders by diet. And isn't that a better and more natural way to live?

A whole new life has opened up to you because you've taken control of your metabolism simply by changing the way you eat. By doing so, you've reprogrammed your body to handle food more efficiently, the way nature intended. As long as you continue to follow low-carb eating principles, as long as you avoid the habits that made you insulin resistant in the first place, your body will continue to burn fat effectively, you'll keep your cholesterol, triglycerides, blood pressure, or blood sugar in normal balance, you'll maintain your lean muscle mass—and taken together, all these things will give you the metabolic staying power to remain healthy and fit for life.

CHAPTER 2

Transition: The Journey Begins

What Are Your Goals in Transition?

The transition phase, as its name suggests, is an interim step between the most carb-restrictive level of the corrective phase and the richer level of maintenance. In the transition phase, you should accomplish the following things:

- You should further stabilize your metabolism.
- You should further improve the sensitivity of your insulin system.
- You should continue to shed the last few pounds you need to lose to finally reach your ideal weight goal.
- You should see further improvement in blood values if they are still slightly abnormal.
- You will make your own meal plan decisions.
- You will cement your results using solid nutritional practices, based on sensible low-carb food principles, which will prepare you for a lifetime of maintenance.

Moving into the Transition Phase

Moving from the corrective phase to the transition phase is easy. All you have to do is eat more. Now that's something you don't often hear on a diet program—eat more! In transition, you'll continue to eat at least your required minimum amount of protein at each meal and choose healthy fats; these foods form the foundation or the base of your maintenance diet. Yet now you'll begin to include more carbohydrate foods, drawing on more and larger servings of the green and colorful vegetables and fruits that should form the lion's share of your carbohydrate intake, but also, if you desire, adding an occasional small serving of the more concentrated carbohydrate foods that were impossible to realistically incorporate at the corrective level—half a banana, for instance, or a small serving of hot cereal (such as a 50/50 blend of steel-cut oats and oat bran) at breakfast. Whereas the total day's carbohydrate intake during the corrective phase of an honest low-carb diet will rarely exceed 30 effective grams per day, the carb allotment in transition will increase to about 15 effective grams per meal, with another optional 5 to 10 grams in a snack, for a daily total of 45 to 55 effective grams per day.[1]

Taking this initial step—slightly increasing the amount of carbohydrates you eat at each meal, from a small serving to a moderate one—will allow your body and your metabolism to adjust gradually and meet the challenge of a higher carbohydrate intake. This adjustment period will help to ensure that you are able to maintain the results you've achieved so far. Some people are very carbohydrate sensitive and won't be able to handle even the transition level increase without losing some ground. That's why it's very important to make this transition gradually, as you carefully monitor your progress. Your commitment and hard work have gotten you this far; now you want to make sure that everything remains stable.

Clifton's Story: A Cautionary Tale

Years ago, we received a long letter from a *Protein Power* reader, Clifton, who lived on the East Coast. As a young man, he'd been an officer in the military and considered himself very fit. He believed that he was in excellent health. In his 30s, however, a routine examination uncovered severe elevations of his cholesterol and triglycerides and an increased risk for heart disease. Subsequent evaluations revealed atherosclerosis, with artery

---

1. While it's important to generally aim for the grams of carb suggested per meal or per day, a couple of grams one way or another won't make an enormous difference—unless it's routinely too much. Don't make yourself crazy trying to hit the gram counts on the nose; just try to get pretty close.

blockages in the arteries serving his heart. He embarked, under his physician's care, on an extremely low-fat, practically vegetarian diet and a vigorous exercise program. Despite these efforts, his lab picture didn't improve, and in due course, he was placed on medications to lower his cholesterol and triglycerides. Still, his disease progressed. During the course of the following decade, he gained 30 or 40 pounds and underwent more than one balloon angioplasty to dilate his narrowed coronary arteries.

In desperation, Clifton began to look elsewhere for help and found *Protein Power*. He read it cover to cover, and the science of it made sense to him; he decided that he had nothing to lose. It was with great trepidation, he wrote, that he abandoned his low-fat, semi-vegetarian diet in favor of our strategy in *Protein Power* which included red meat, eggs, cheese, and butter, yet forbade the two-bagel breakfasts, baked potato lunches, and pasta suppers that had been his mainstay for years. With his fingers crossed, he embarked on his new plan and, lo and behold, in six weeks, his numbers had improved. In twelve weeks, they were normal for the first time in more than a decade, and he'd lost 30 pounds. He was so delighted that he just had to write us a letter telling his amazing story.

He felt, and we agreed, that he was ready to make the transition to a maintenance level diet. Following the instructions in our book, he began to increase his carb allotment, slowly at first, then with a little more vigor, until he was eating about 90 grams of effective carbs per day. As we recommend, he asked his doctor to check his blood levels and was shocked to discover that his cholesterol and triglycerides had begun to climb again. He hadn't regained any weight yet, and he felt great, but the numbers worried him. He contacted our office again.

We advised him to return to the corrective level of the diet, remain there for a month, and then repeat the lab tests, which he did. His numbers returned to normal. Based on this response, we felt sure that he was a person who was extremely sensitive to carbohydrates. He might be able to tolerate a slight increase above correction, but probably not much. We recommended that he carefully seek that number by increasing his intake very, very slowly to 45 grams a day for a month, and then to recheck the labs. If all remained stable, he should increase to 50, then 55, then 60 over several months and recheck the labs. At the first sign of higher cholesterol and triglycerides, he should fall back to the last level of carb intake at which his lab values remained in control and call it a day. He adopted that strategy and learned to eat within the limits of his own metabolism.

The moral to the story is this: there is no magic one-size-fits-all maintenance carb number. In transition and maintenance, you can advance your intake of carbs only to the point at which you begin to lose metabolic control, as demonstrated by weight regain, fluid retention, the return of GE reflux symptoms, sleep apnea, inflammatory aches and pains, or changes in lab values. When you reach that point, wherever it is, even if it's at the first step of transition, stop there or your maintenance will unravel. And if that's how it shakes out, so be it. You'll still be able to eat a richly satisfying, healthy selection of foods.

Let's take a look now at what a transition level carb allotment will translate to in meals.

Creating Transition Meals

Let's talk first about quality versus quantity. Although metabolically speaking, in absolute grams a carb is a carb is a carb, clearly all foods containing carbohydrate are not created equal when it comes to their nutrient density. For instance, there are about an equal number of effective carbohydrate grams in a medium tomato and in a teaspoon of table sugar, but there the similarities end. In the tomato, you'll also get 1.5 grams of fiber, 766 IU of vitamin A, 23 mg of vitamin C, 273 mg of potassium, and 14 mg of magnesium, in addition to cancer fighters such as lycopene. In the teaspoon of sugar, you'll get a teaspoon of sugar, nothing but 100 percent pure empty carbohydrates. That's why, as you move into the transition phase, we encourage you to make your added carb allotment count for something. For the most part, you should enjoy bigger servings of colorful fruits and vegetables and the gradual return of small servingsof starchier foods, such as beans, peas, and yams, with the addition of occasional small servings of whole grains, such as wild rice or steel-cut oats.

By now, you should be well acquainted with the corrective phase meals that enabled you to lose weight and restore your metabolic machinery, having eaten those kinds of meals regularly as you completed the first leg of your low-carb journey toward a leaner, healthier body.[2] To help you ease into transition, we've provided several days of dual purpose meal plans, with each meal designed to be suitable for either the corrective or the transition level. These meal plans will serve as an illustrative template that compares what you can eat in correction with what you'll enjoy in transition; you'll quickly see that the only difference between them is a slightly larger serving of carbohydrate foods in transition. We've shown in italics the food additions that turn a corrective level meal into a transition meal. You may wish to use these corrective level meal plans a time or two each to solidify your corrected position and ensure that you actually start out at a corrective carb level. If you've been a bit lax in monitoring your carb intake lately—a phenomenon not uncommon to long-term low-carb dieters—you may be surprised to find yourself losing a pound or two after you had been stable or stalled. You can then repeat these meals with the transition level additions and move ahead from there.

In designing our meal plans, we strove to minimize the time you spend preparing meals. Since it takes no longer to cook two chicken breasts than it does three, for instance, you can make each meal do double duty by cooking a bit extra, so that it's ready for lunch the next day. In most cases, one night's dinner becomes the next day's lunch, so look ahead to future meals. We've also tried to strike a balance between variety and common sense; instead of a different fruit or vegetable at every meal, you can use the same fresh fruits and vegetables for several meals in a row.

These meals are general guidelines. You'll notice that while we give specific amounts of the carbohydrate portion of your meal—that is, the fruits, the veggies, and the bread—we don't specify how much protein you'll eat. That's because while carbohydrate allotment remains the same for everyone in correction or in transition, the protein serving varies from one person to another. It depends on your height, weight, and gender (among other things) and is specified in the Protein Requirements for men and women in appendix A. Select the serving size that meets your protein requirement, of whatever protein food the meal plan specifies— be that chicken, fish, beef, or eggs—and do the same for each person you cook or buy for. Be sure to allow enough extra for tomorrow's meal, too.

2. If you're unfamiliar with corrective level meals and would like some guidance, we refer you to our *30-Day Low-Carb Diet Solution,* where you'll find a full month of corrective breakfasts, lunches, dinners, and snacks, as well as nearly a hundred recipes.

One final word about the meal plans in this book: it's okay if you don't cook. Although we strongly feel that the most certain road to long-term success on a low-carb diet (or on any diet, for that matter) goes straight through the kitchen, it's not the only road. The most obvious advantage of cooking—aside from the economic one—is quality: if you make it yourself, you know what's in it. Hidden sugars, starches, or unhealthy fats won't sandbag you. But more important, we believe that you can't fully embrace dietary change and make it part of your life for good until you begin to eat—and cook—that way for yourself. If you don't have time to cook, don't want to cook, don't know how to cook, and have no desire to learn, fine. You can certainly purchase similar suitable foods already prepared from deli counters, hot tables, salad bars, or restaurants. Use common sense to make reasonable substitutions to the meal plans, if necessary. Whether you make it yourself or buy it already made, here's what it should generally look like.

A Tale of Two Levels: Corrective Meals Compared to Transition Meals

Day 1

BREAKFAST   Poached eggs and sausage
            1 slice low-carb toast, buttered
            ½ cup fresh or frozen strawberries
            Transition addition: 1 fresh tomato, sliced

LUNCH   Tuna salad–stuffed tomato (cut a whole tomato in wedges
               partly through, fan the wedges into a star, fill with tuna
               salad, and dress with olive oil vinaigrette)
            3 or 4 Blue Diamond Nut Thin[3] crackers with butter
            Transition addition: ½ cup grapes

SNACK   Hard salami and cheese slices (1–2 ounces each) and
               ⅓ cup grapes
            Transition addition: 4 or 5 Blue Diamond Nut Thin crackers

DINNER   Baked or grilled herbed chicken breasts (rub with olive oil
               and sprinkle with salt, pepper, garlic powder, and rose-
               mary)

3. Blue Diamond Nut Thin crackers are available at most natural food retailers and grocery stores nationwide; ask your grocer. They contain 1.4 grams of effective carbs per cracker.

½ cup green beans

Salad greens with choice of low-carb dressing

½ cup fresh or frozen strawberries with whipped cream if
desired

Transition addition: ½ cup more green beans

Day 2

BREAKFAST   Hi-Protein Yogurt (mix ½ cup plain yogurt, 1–2 scoops
low-carb protein powder, and 1 packet Splenda; top
with 1 tablespoon sliced almonds)
Transition addition: ½ cup mixed berries

LUNCH   Grilled chicken wrap (leftover chicken in a low-carb
tortilla, with lettuce, tomato, onion, sprouts, mayo,
mustard, and 1 slice of cheese, as desired)
Green salad with choice of dressing
Transition addition: ½ cup cantaloupe

SNACK   Hardboiled or deviled egg(s) and ½ orange
Transition addition: ½ orange (for a total of 1 orange)

DINNER   Grilled or broiled salmon (or other firm-fleshed fish)
10 spears fresh asparagus, steamed, roasted, or sautéed in
olive oil
Green salad with raw broccoli, cauliflower, sprouts, and
choice of dressing
½ fresh peach, sliced, with a dollop of whipped cream
*Transition addition: ½ cup beets, with salt, pepper, and
butter*

Day 3

BREAKFAST   Ham and cheese omelet
Berry slush (in the blender, puree ½ cup frozen unsweetened mixed berries, ½ cup water, 1 packet Splenda)
5 spears cooked fresh asparagus
Transition addition: 1 slice low-carb toast, buttered

LUNCH   Salmon chef salad (romaine, salmon, hardboiled egg
wedges, black olives, 1 fresh tomato, ½ cup raw
broccoli/cauliflower, with dressing of choice)

*Transition addition: low-carb croutons (made of 1 slice
   low-carb bread, buttered, sprinkled with garlic salt,
   cubed, and toasted)*

SNACK   1–2 ounces dry roasted or raw almonds and ½ small apple
*Transition addition: ½ small apple (for a total of 1 small
   apple)*

DINNER   Grilled or broiled steak or burger
½ cup sautéed zucchini (or other summer squash)
½ cup stewed tomatoes
Salad greens with choice of dressing
*Transition addition: ½ fresh peach with a dollop of
   whipped cream*

It's very easy to create your own transition meals. One way to approach transition meal planning is to take favorite meals from the corrective phase of your low-carb diet and simply add a small serving of another carbohydrate food (from the Carbohydrate Servings Lists in appendix B) to the meal. Or, you can start from scratch, pairing a healthy (and appropriate) serving of meat, fish, seafood, eggs, or poultry with the small and moderate carbohydrate servings from your list.

Here's how to do it using the Meal Planner Worksheet you'll find in appendix C:

- Select a protein food to be the cornerstone of your meal. (Remember that you may need to adjust your protein serving size based on your height and your new lower weight, using the Protein Requirements charts for men and women in appendix A. Find your correct protein serving size in the Protein Servings Lists in appendix B and write it on the worksheet.)

- Select the carb portion of your meal. What fruit, veggie, or bread and cereal grain items from the carbohydrate servings lists would you like to accompany your protein cornerstone? In transition, you have the choice of two moderate carbohydrate servings or, if you prefer, three selections from the small servings list for even greater variety.

Here's an example of what a completed meal plan worksheet might look like:

Meal Planner Worksheet

Protein Serving Size   _____L_____ (S, M, L, XL, XXL)

Carbohydrate Serving Size ___moderate___ (small, moderate, large)

	Yes	No
Did you take your multivitamin/mineral?	☑	☐
Did you take extra potassium/magnesium?	☑	☐

What you plan to eat

Breakfast:

Protein serving — Bacon cheddar omelet (3 eggs + 1 ounce cheese + 2 strips bacon)

Carb serving — 1 slice buttered low-carb toast

½ small banana

Fluid (ounces) — 8 ounces coffee with cream and 8 ounces water

Lunch:

Protein serving — 2 broiled salmon burgers

Carb serving — spinach salad with 2 cups fresh spinach, ½ cup fresh mushroom slices, ½ cup chopped spring onions, ½ cup shredded carrots, 2 slices crisp crumbled bacon and blue cheese dressing.

½ cup fresh strawberries for dessert

Fluid (ounces) — 16 ounces iced tea, sweetened with Splenda

Snack: — 1 ounce hard salami slices, 1 ounce cheddar cheese on 6 Blue Diamond Nut Thin crackers with mustard

½ cup grapes

12 ounces mineral water

Dinner:

Protein serving — 6 ounces grilled flank steak with herbed butter

Carb serving — 1 large zucchini, sautéed in olive oil with ¼ onion, 1 clove garlic, and 4 cherry tomato halves.

1 large green salad with ½ tomato and ranch dressing

1 ounce commercial low-carb chocolate

Fluid (ounces) — 3 ounces dry red wine

8 ounces water, 6 ounces decaf coffee with cream

Using one of your blank meal planner worksheets and your Protein and Carbohydrate Servings Lists, practice building a few transition level meals on your own, based on the foods you prefer. (Before using it, make additional copies of the worksheet.) You may wonder why you even need these meal planner work sheets, when you have a 365-day journal. The two serve different purposes: your meal planner worksheets are there for you to use as a learning exercise, for planning what you *will* eat. Your journal should be an honest record of what you *did* eat. By planning in advance and keeping careful records in your journal, you'll soon get a good feel for the amounts of the various kinds of fruits, veggies, and bread and cereal grain products that are suitable for this stage of your program. Then you'll be well on your way to learning to live low carb for life.

Planning Your Transition Snacks

Although you may not feel as pressing a need to snack now that you've completed the corrective phase and are moving into transition, there will still be times when a mid-morning or mid-afternoon snack will be helpful to keep you from getting hungry and diving into the wrong sort of food. The rule of keeping good, healthy snacks at the ready isn't just for the first phase of your program; it's a good idea at any time.

Just as has happened with your meals, the carbohydrate serving for your snacks can increase a bit now, too—it doesn't have to, but it *can*. In planning a snack, you can use the following rule of thumb: eat an amount of protein equal to about one-third to one-half of your required protein serving for meals. For instance, if your serving size of meat is small or medium (3 or 4 ounces), a good snack size for protein would be about 1 or 2 ounces of meat or meat and cheese combined. If your serving requirement is large or extra-large (about 5 or 6 ounces), a good snack size would be about 2 or 3 ounces of meat or meat and cheese.

If you're having an especially hungry day for some reason, it's certainly fine to eat a bit more protein, but remember, this is a snack, not a meal. Dinner is on the way soon enough. Remember, too, that snacking is an option. You certainly don't have to have a snack every day or snack at all if you feel satisfied by your three meals; it's just nice to know that you can and nice to be prepared with good choices at your disposal if you choose to indulge.

Along with the protein in your snacks, your expanded carbohydrate allotment—you can enjoy two small servings now—will allow you to have a number of whole fruits, such as a small peach or a plum, a whole kiwi, a tangerine, or even half of a banana, apple, or pear. In the veggie world, you can enjoy an almost limitless amount of crunchy raw fibrous veggies, such as broccoli, cauliflower, radishes, celery, and even a respectable portion of raw carrots. So how about snacking on a little leftover steak or chicken with a fresh peach or with raw veggies and some healthy blue cheese dressing for dipping?

How Long Do You Stay in Transition?

Your stay in this phase of the diet depends on the kind of issues you were addressing at the start. If your only concern was weight, you can spend as little as two weeks in transition, and if your weight remains stable, you can move into maintenance; don't worry, though, there's no hard and fast rule that says you must move on at a certain time. If you'd like to stay at this level for several more weeks of consolidation to get your feet solidly under you in this less-carbohydrate-restrictive phase, that's fine.

If correcting health issues such as elevated cholesterol, triglycerides, blood sugar, or blood pressure was among your original goals, then we'd recommend that you plan to stay in transition for at least a month to allow your blood values to stabilize at this new higher-carb level. After at least four weeks at this slightly higher carbohydrate intake, we suggest that you see your physician to repeat any necessary laboratory tests. It's perfectly fine for you to remain in transition for several months if you feel comfortable at that level and want to postpone getting the repeat laboratory tests and moving ahead. If, in the transition phase, your cholesterol, triglycerides, blood sugar, and/or blood pressure remain stable, then you'll be ready to move on to the maintenance phase.

Keep Those Fluids Coming!

You'll notice that in the following meal plans, we have not specified any beverages. That's not because you shouldn't still drink plenty of fluids;

you should continue to try to drink 64 ounces of water or noncaloric fluids every day. Rather, it's because we want to give you freedom of choice. You could drink water; black, green, white, herbal, or decaffeinated tea; regular or decaffeinated coffee; or diet sodas sweetened with Splenda, acesulfame-K, stevia, or saccharine (not with aspartame because of health concerns). And, of course, you could continue to have a small (3 to 4 ounces) glass of dry red or white wine or a 12-ounce light or low-carb beer for about 3 or 4 carbohydrate grams if you desire. Enjoy, but remember that beer and wine do contribute to your daily carb and calorie intake, so don't go overboard.

A Word to Vegetarians

The following meal plans were designed for an omnivorous palate and include not only eggs and dairy, but meat, poultry, and fish as well. If you will eat fish but are not crazy about other meats, you may substitute any of the fish dishes for the beef, lamb, pork, or chicken dishes you cannot eat. In other cases, you can simply substitute a soy-based or TVP alternative—for instance, veggie burger for lamb burger or hamburger, veggie bacon for pork, veggie breakfast links for sausage, veggie hot dogs or lunch "meats" for deli meats—with a modest increase in total carb content. You'll find a number of vegetarian recipes in our *30-Day Low-Carb Diet Solution* and on our Web site (www.proteinpower.com). On the Web site's bulletin board, you'll find a forum that includes other low-carbing vegetarians, admittedly not a large community. If you discover wonderful ideas for low-carb vegetarian dishes that you'd like to share with others, you may do so there.

Transition Phase Meal Plans

These meal plans are interchangeable—feel free to exchange any breakfast for another breakfast, any lunch for a lunch, a snack for a snack, or a dinner for a dinner if you can't or won't eat a particular food, don't have the ingredients on hand, or are dining away from home with limited choices. If you don't cook and want a really simple plan, you can use the generic ultra-easy meal plan, as follows:

Generic Transition Level Meal Plan

BREAKFAST   Eggs any style, with bacon, ham, sausage, or fish, if desired
1 slice low-carb toast with butter
½ cup melon or berries or ½ piece of fruit

LUNCH   Bacon cheeseburger or grilled chicken breast "protein
style" (that's sans bun and wrapped in two large lettuce
leaves)
Salad greens with tomato wedges, raw broccoli, cauliflower,
and mushrooms as desired and choice of dressing
1 peach, plum, or tangerine or ½ cup grapes

SNACK   1 peach, plum, or tangerine or ½ cup grapes
1–2 ounces raw or dry roasted nuts or deli meat or hard
cheese

DINNER   Grilled/broiled steak, chicken, or fish
1 cup green or colorful low-starch vegetable
Salad greens with tomato wedges, raw veggies, and
dressing
½ cup berries or melon

Two Weeks of Customized Transition Level Meal Plans

Day 1

BREAKFAST   Scrambled eggs and sausage in a low-carb tortilla with salsa
1 cup mixed berries, fresh or frozen

LUNCH   Chef salad (extra meat and cheese for M, L, XL, XXL)
4 Blue Diamond Nut Thin Crackers[4] or 1 low carb-tortilla

SNACK   1 peach and 1–2 ounces cheddar cheese

DINNER   Baked chicken
½ cup eggplant, sautéed in olive oil with 1 tablespoon
chopped onion and ¼ cup diced canned tomatoes,
topped with grated Parmesan cheese

---

4. Blue Diamond Nut Thin crackers are available at most natural food retailers and grocery stores nationwide; ask your grocer. They contain 1.4 grams of effective carbs per cracker.

Green salad with olive oil vinaigrette

Sauteed asparagus (about 6 to 8 spears) with butter

½ cup commercial low-carb ice cream (select one with 4 or fewer grams of sugar alcohol per serving to limit gastrointestinal side effects)

Day 2

BREAKFAST Protein fruit smoothie (blend 1 cup frozen mixed berries, 1 serving vanilla protein powder, ½ cup plain yogurt, ½ cup water, and 1 packet Splenda)

1 slice low-carb toast, buttered

LUNCH Roasted chicken wrap (leftover chicken in a low-carb tortilla dressed with fresh spinach, avocado, tomato, onion, mayo, and mustard)

½ cup grapes

SNACK 1 ounce hard salami, 1 ounce cheddar cheese, and 1 tangerine

DINNER Grilled salmon

Grilled asparagus spears (6 to 8)

Sliced fresh tomato drizzled with olive oil and balsamic vinegar

Sliced fresh peach with cream (or ½ cup frozen, unsweetened peaches)

Day 3

BREAKFAST Cottage cheese

½ cup berries, fresh or frozen

Crisp bacon

1 slice low-carb toast, buttered

LUNCH Salmon Caesar salad (romaine, leftover grilled salmon, Caesar dressing)

4 to 6 Blue Diamond Nut Thin Crackers or 2 to 3 fat-free saltines with butter

½ apple

SNACK 1–2 ounces almonds and ½ apple

DINNER Grilled lamb burgers (or hamburgers)

1 cup stewed canned tomatoes

Salad greens and ½ cup raw veggies (broccoli, cauliflower, carrot) with minted yogurt dressing (1 tablespoon plain yogurt, 1 teaspoon heavy cream, 1 teaspoon finely chopped mint leaves, salt, and pepper)

½ cup commercial low-carb ice cream (if desired) (select one with 4 or fewer grams of sugar alcohol per serving to limit gastrointestinal side effects)

Day 4

BREAKFAST Ham and cheese omelet

½ cup melon (fresh or frozen)

½ medium tomato, sliced

1 warm low-carb tortilla with butter and 1 teaspoon low-carb jam

LUNCH Lamb burger wrap (leftover burger wrapped in a low-carb tortilla with fresh spinach, onion, tomato, and minted yogurt dressing)

1 tangerine

SNACK 6 Blue Diamond Nut Thins (or 3 fat-free saltines) with 2 tablespoons peanut or almond butter

DINNER Pork roast or tenderloin

1 cup buttered brussels sprouts, sprinkled with salt, pepper, and garlic powder

1 medium tomato, in wedges, with Roquefort dressing

½ cup commercial low-carb ice cream (if desired) (select one with 4 or fewer grams of sugar alcohol per serving to limit gastrointestinal side effects)

Day 5

BREAKFAST Hi-Pro Yogurt (8 ounces plain yogurt plus 1 serving flavored low-carb protein powder)

LUNCH Pork pita pocket (heat chopped pork roast or tenderloin, 1 ounce low-carb barbecue sauce, and 1 tablespoon chopped onion, and stuff into ½ small pita pocket lined with a large lettuce leaf)

½ cup coleslaw (no sugar added)

SNACK   1 tangerine and 1–2 ounces string cheese

DINNER   Baked fish, drizzled with olive oil, salt, pepper, herbs, and
                    a squeeze of lemon
                ½ cup broccoli, sautéed in olive oil and garlic
                ½ red, green, or yellow bell pepper, sautéed or roasted
                    alongside fish
                1 medium tomato, wedged, topped with blue cheese
                    dressing and 1 ounce blue cheese crumbles
                ½ cup fresh or frozen berries, dollop of whipped cream

Day 6

BREAKFAST   Omelet with cheese and bacon
                ½ cup leftover sautéed broccoli
                1 low-carb tortilla, warmed, with butter and 1 teaspoon
                    low-carb jam
                ½ cup fresh or frozen melon

LUNCH   2 fish soft tacos (leftover baked fish, warmed, wrapped in
                    warm low-carb tortillas with shredded lettuce, diced
                    tomato, and homemade mayonnaise spiced with a dash
                    of cumin and chili powder)
                1 medium Valencia orange or tangerine

SNACK   1–2 ounces nuts and 1 cup grapes

DINNER   Rotisserie chicken
                ⅓ cup canned butter beans
                Green salad with tomato wedges and good olive oil dressing
                ½ cup commercial low-carb ice cream (if desired) (select
                    one with 4 or fewer grams of sugar alcohol per serving
                    to limit gastrointestinal side effects)

Day 7

BREAKFAST   Protein fruit smoothie (see *Day 2*)

LUNCH   Bacon cheeseburger, "protein style"[5] or top bun removed,
                    with tomato, avocado, onion, mayo, mustard, and pickle
                    as desired

---

5. More and more restaurants will wrap your burger or chicken sandwich in two large lettuce
leaves on request. In-N-Out Burger calls this option "protein style"; we approve.

Green salad with choice of low-carb dressing (add ¾ cup
raw veggies if you remove both buns)
1 medium plum or peach

SNACK 1–2 ounces hard salami, 1–2 ounces hard cheese, 1 cup
grapes
1 cup tomato bisque (or any clear broth or creamy soup
without noodles or potatoes)

DINNER 1–2 slices quiche Lorraine (or your favorite) without crust
(XL, XXL protein servings, add 1 or 2 pieces rotisserie
chicken for added protein)
1 green salad with at least ½ cup raw veggies (broccoli,
cauliflower, and carrots) and choice of dressing
2 small squares (about 1 ounce) commercial low-carb
chocolate bar (if desired)

Day 8

BREAKFAST Fruit and cream burrito (fill two warm low-carb tortillas
with a mixture of ¼ cup cottage cheese, ¼ cup plain
yogurt, 1 serving strawberry protein powder, and
¼ cup mixed berries (fresh or frozen) and 1–2 packets
Splenda)

LUNCH Tuna salad sandwich (tuna salad on 2 slices low-carb bread,
with lettuce, mayo, mustard, and pickle as desired)
Green salad with tomatoes, mushrooms, beets, cheese,
and good dressing

SNACK 1 cup each fresh broccoli and cauliflower florets with
2 ounces ranch or blue cheese dressing

DINNER Grilled or broiled steak
¾ cup cooked carrots (buttered, if desired)
The Wedge (iceberg lettuce wedge, topped with blue
cheese dressing, blue cheese and bacon crumbles, and
diced tomato)
1 cup sliced fresh or frozen strawberries sweetened with
Splenda

Day 9

BREAKFAST   Low-carb French toast (soak 2 slices low-carb bread in a
                    mixture of 1 beaten egg, 2 tablespoons cream, and a
                    pinch of nutmeg; fry in butter until set)
                ¼ cup commercial low-carb syrup
                Link or patty sausage
                ½ cup fresh or frozen blueberries

LUNCH   Steak wrap (leftover steak in a warm low-carb tortilla with
                    fresh spinach, sliced tomato, onion, pickles, mayo, and
                    mustard as desired)
                1 tangerine or small orange or ½ cup grapes

SNACK   2 to 4 deli roll-ups (thin beef or ham slices, thin cheese
                    slices, a spread of mustard or horseradish; roll and
                    secure with toothpicks) and 1 cup grapes

DINNER   Grilled or broiled salmon (or other fish)
                10 spears steamed, sautéed, or roasted asparagus, topped
                    with olive oil and sprinkled with Parmesan cheese and a
                    bit of garlic powder)
                ¾ cup boiled or roasted beets
                Green salad with tomato wedges and good low-carb
                    dressing
                1 slice low-carb garlic toast (toasted low-carb bread, but-
                    tered, and sprinkled garlic powder)
                ½ cup commercial low-carb ice cream (if desired) (select
                    one with 4 or fewer grams of sugar alcohol per serving
                    to limit gastrointestinal side effects)

Day 10

BREAKFAST   Veggie and cheese omelet (made with sautéed broccoli,
                    garlic, onion, tomato, and cheese)
                2 small low-carb tortillas, warm, with butter and low-carb
                    jam
                1 cup fresh or frozen melon

LUNCH   Salmon Caesar salad (romaine, leftover fish, Caesar
                    dressing, Parmesan cheese)

1 slice low-carb garlic toast as croutons (cut low-carb
bread into small squares, toast in broiler, toss with
melted butter mixed with a sprinkle of garlic powder)
1 fresh peach (or ½ cup unsweetened frozen sliced
peaches)

SNACK Hard salami chips (place 1–2 ounces thin salami slices,
sprinkled with Parmesan cheese, on several layers of
paper toweling and microwave for 1 to 1½ minutes until
crunchy) and 1 tangerine

DINNER Grilled or broiled bratwurst
¾ cup sauerkraut
½ cup applesauce
Green salad with raw broccoli/cauliflower and choice of
low-carb dressing

Day 11

BREAKFAST Protein fruit smoothie (see *Day 2*)
Bacon or sausage

LUNCH Brat and mustard wrap (split leftover brat in warm
low-carb tortilla with fresh spinach, tomato, onion,
pickle, and mustard as desired)
1 tangerine

SNACK 6 to 8 Blue Diamond Nut Thin crackers with 2 tablespoons
almond or low-sugar peanut butter

DINNER Grilled or sautéed shrimp
1 cup cooked spaghetti squash (or other summer squash
variety), dressed with butter, salt, pepper, and Parmesan
cheese
Green salad with a wedged tomato, sprouts, raw veggies,
and choice of dressing
1 slice low-carb garlic toast (low-carb bread, butter, sprinkled with garlic powder)
½ cup commercial low-carb ice cream (if desired) (select
one with 4 or fewer grams of sugar alcohol per serving
to limit gastrointestinal side effects)

Day 12

BREAKFAST   Eggs any style with Canadian bacon
1 cup fresh or frozen mixed berries
1 slice low-carb toast with butter and low-carb jam

LUNCH   Chef salad with shrimp (use leftover shrimp in place of
other meat alongside boiled eggs, fresh veggies, and
cheese)
Your choice of low-carb dressing
6 Blue Diamond Nut Thin crackers with butter

SNACK   2 ounces beef jerky and 1 cup grapes

DINNER   Baked, broiled, or grilled fish
1 cup sautéed red or yellow bell peppers
1 cup steamed brussels sprouts, dressed with butter, salt,
and pepper
½ cup low-carb ice cream (if desired) (select one with
4 or fewer grams of sugar alcohol per serving to limit
gastrointestinal side effects)

Day 13

BREAKFAST   Hi-Pro Yogurt (see *Day 2*)

LUNCH   2 fish soft tacos (leftover fish and peppers in warm
low-carb tortillas with shredded lettuce or cabbage,
diced tomatoes, and fresh parsley or cilantro. Dress with
homemade mayo[6] spiced with a dash of cumin and chili
powder and a squeeze of fresh lime juice.)
1 tangerine

SNACK   1–2 ounces deli meat with 1–2 cups raw broccoli and
cauliflower and ranch dressing

DINNER   Pork roast or tenderloin

---

6. Making your own mayonnaise lets you control the quality of the oil you use, which is important to your health. A bit of commercial mayonnaise won't hurt you, but if you're fond of this
condiment, learn to make your own. You'll find recipes for homemade mayonnaise in our
30-Day Low-Carb Diet Solution, in *The Low-Carb Comfort Food Cookbook,* and on our Web
site, www.proteinpower.com or www.lowcarbcookworx.com.

1 zucchini or yellow squash sautéed in olive oil with garlic, salt, and pepper

Sliced fresh tomato with slices of mozzarella cheese, drizzled with olive oil and balsamic vinegar

½ cup applesauce

Day 14

BREAKFAST   2 poached eggs, each on ½ slice low-carb buttered toast and 1 slice Canadian bacon (XL and XXL, add extra bacon)

4 or 5 spears steamed fresh asparagus spears (with hollandaise sauce, if desired)

1 cup strawberries, fresh or frozen

LUNCH   BBQ pork wrap (leftover tenderloin with low-carb commercial BBQ sauce, lettuce, tomato, onion, and pickle as desired)

½ cup coleslaw (no sugar added)

½ apple

SNACK   1 ounce hard salami, 1 ounce hard cheese, ½ apple

DINNER   Grilled hamburger

1½ cups green beans

¼ cup corn

Salad greens with good olive oil dressing

½ cup strawberries (fresh or frozen) with whipped cream

What Next?

You've now completed the first two weeks of the transition period. Take a moment to assess your current state of health and fitness about the issues that you solved during the corrective phase. Since moving to transition. . . .

	Week 2		Week 4	
	Yes	No	Yes	No
Has your weight increased?	☐	☐	☐	☐
Has your waist size increased?	☐	☐	☐	☐
Has your blood pressure gone up?	☐	☐	☐	☐

	Week 2		Week 4	
	Yes	No	Yes	No
Are your rings or shoes tighter from fluid?	☐	☐	☐	☐
Are you experiencing heartburn?	☐	☐	☐	☐

(After week 4, please answer the following questions as well.)

	Yes	No
Has your blood sugar risen above normal?	☐	☐
Has your insulin risen above normal?	☐	☐
Have your triglycerides increased above normal?	☐	☐

If you have answered no to the first five questions, you are tolerating the added carbohydrates well and can generally expect to remain stable at this level of carb intake. For now, you may either repeat the fourteen days of transition meals or, better yet, begin creating your own transition level meals using the Carbohydrate Servings Lists and your imagination. After two more weeks in transition, answer the same set of questions again, this time with the laboratory measurements.[7] If you were able to answer no to all questions, your target lab values and readings are normal, and you feel ready to do so, you can begin slowly to increase your carb servings toward your final maintenance level.

If you have answered yes to any question, you should return to the corrective level of carb intake and spend a couple of weeks stabilizing there again; allow your weight and any abnormal lab measurements to drop once more to their pretransition levels. Once you've accomplished this, try again to increase your carbohydrates to the transition level. If once again you find that you begin to lose ground, you may already be near your carb-tolerance point. To inch up a bit farther, try eating a moderate carbohydrate serving at breakfast and servings from the small carbohydrate list the remainder of the day. If you tolerate this much, try moderate servings at breakfast and lunch, but keep the snack and the dinner carbohydrate intakes at the smaller level.

7. Only people whose levels were elevated initially must check blood work at this point; however, it's certainly a good idea for everyone. Diabetic patients accustomed to self-monitoring their blood sugar should check sugars daily as they increase their carbohydrate intake. Be sure to record your results in your journal.

Like our patient Clifton, whose story you read earlier, some people's metabolisms are quite sensitive to carbohydrates, and they are unable to increase their intake much beyond 40 to 50 effective grams a day without seeing some evidence of metabolic impact, such as weight gain, fluid retention, the return of GE reflux and heartburn, elevations in blood pressure, or increases in blood levels of triglycerides or blood sugar. For these individuals, long-term maintenance of weight and good health demand that they keep pretty tight control of their carbohydrate intake over the long haul. For these people, if weight continues to decline, the calories needed to maintain weight should come from lean protein and good-quality fats—things such as lean meats and fish, nuts, nut butters, olives, avocados, eggs, and cheese—instead of from additional sources of more concentrated carbohydrates. It is especially important if you are in this group to make the carbs you eat count nutritionally; be sure to eat a wide variety of fibrous green and colorful vegetables and low-sugar fruits for the bulk of your daily carb intake. Most of the time, try to steer clear of concentrated sources of carbohydrates—the starchier fruits and veggies such as potatoes, bananas and other tropical fruits, and wheat, oats, corn, rice, and other cereal grains—that will take up a big portion of your carb allotment for little nutritional gain.

For most people, the additional carbohydrate servings of transition present no problem in their maintaining optimal metabolic balance; they will be able to tolerate even greater intake as they move ahead into the maintenance phase of the plan.

Don't be disheartened if you fall into the more sensitive category. We're all different; some of us are simply less tolerant of carbohydrates than others are, but each of us will tolerate enough to make for a rich and satisfying carb-controlled diet over the long term.

In fact, just as there's no one-size-fits-all tolerable number of carb grams, there's not even a magic number specific to you that will hold true in all situations forever. The number of carb grams you will tolerate in maintenance is both unique to you and dependent on your lifestyle at a given point in time. What you'll tolerate while in training for the Ironman will be higher than what you'll tolerate if you're laid up with a broken leg—we'd be remiss in not pointing that out. There is a very real activity part of the weight and health maintenance equation: the more active you are, the more carbohydrates you'll tolerate in maintenance, and its obvious corollary—the less active you are, the less you'll tolerate. We'll take a closer look at that connection in the next chapter. In the meantime, if you're having trouble advancing past the transition level and you'd like to be able to eat a somewhat higher-carb diet and stay in control, try increasing your level of physical activity if you're able to—lift weights, hike, bike, dance, swim, ski, or play tennis, golf, basketball, hockey, or whatever you enjoy doing. After a month or so, take another Progress Chart to see what effect the added activity has on your weight and lab values.

You may find that you're able to eat a few more carbs or you may confirm that you've already reached your limit. But it doesn't really matter what number of carbs you're able to eat and still maintain. Your challenges are the same: learning to live in balance and harmony with your own metabolism, recognizing that maintenance is not a destination but a journey, learning how to adjust your plan as needed to cope with changing life situations, and identifying those situations when they arise. We'll tackle these topics in the next chapters.

CHAPTER 3

Maintenance: One Size Fits You

Now the journey continues, toward what will become your maximum carbohydrate allotment for maintenance. You may find it within the next week or two; in fact, for many people that will be the case. For some people, particularly those who are very physically active, it may take a month or longer. We hasten to remind you that the absolute number is not as important as the principle: you will successfully maintain your weight or health only by keeping your daily effective carb intake at or below the level that your metabolism will tolerate *at a given time and a given level of activity.* This number may change as your circumstances change, and you must learn to be flexible. For now, you're seeking to determine a benchmark.

To guide you along the way, we've designed a series of meal plans that gradually increases your carb load week by week. For Week 1, you'll find three meal plans that provide a large carbohydrate serving at breakfast and moderate carb servings at lunch, dinner, and a snack. You may repeat these meal plans over the course of the first week or create your own using the Carbohydrate Servings Lists. Recall that your carb serving at any level consists of any two choices from the list for that level; for instance, a moderate serving of carbohydrates at a meal could be a moderate serving of a vegetable plus either a moderate serving of fruit or an item from the moderate bread and cereal grain category. It could also be two fruit servings or two vegetable servings or even half servings of four different items, if you'd like.

At the end of the first week, assess your state of health and fitness, and if everything has remained stable with weight and health measures, you can advance to Week 2. Take care not to push your intake beyond your limits; if your control begins to slip on the higher level of carbs, back up a notch and stay there. If you find that you've reached your carb limit in this first week of maintenance, that's fine. It's important to remember that you should not advance to a higher carb intake if you see that you're beginning to lose control of your weight or health; stop where you're stable. If you stay at the Week 1 level, you'll want to begin constructing your own meals around this pattern: a moderate serving of carbohydrates at breakfast, lunch, and dinner, and a small to moderate one as an optional snack. Following this pattern, your daily carb allotment should be roughly 50 to 60 effective carb grams a day. Don't stress over trying to hit a number on the nose; just get into that ballpark most of the time, which you'll easily do by taking your cues from the serving sizes suggested in the Carbohydrate Servings Lists in appendix B.

If you're moving on, follow the Week 2 meal plans; you'll be eating about 65 to 70 grams of effective carbohydrates divided as a large carbohydrate serving at breakfast and lunch and a moderate one for dinner and a snack. Repeat them as necessary for at least one week and reassess. If you have no weight gain and no deterioration of health or lab readings, you can move to Week 3, where meals include large servings at all three meals and a moderate snack serving. The Week 3 level meals will provide about 80 grams of effective carbs per day.

Reassess at the end of the week, and if you find that you're still able to increase without losing control, move to Week 4, where all meals and snacks contain large carbohydrate servings, providing about 90 to 95 grams of effective carbohydrates per day. Few people outside of serious competitive athletes will have the carbohydrate tolerance to move much beyond the fourth week, but if you remain stable after Week 4, and you'd still like more to eat, you can increase your breakfast by an additional small carb serving for another week. If you remain stable for a week, increase your lunch, then your dinner, then your snack at weekly intervals. You may stop increasing at any time; if you're satisfied with the amounts you're eating and you're not still losing weight, there's no reason to move on. You don't have to stuff yourself. Always stop eating when you're full and satisfied.

The Maintenance Meal Plans

Week 1

Day 1

BREAKFAST Ham and cheese omelet
½ banana
½ cup fresh or frozen blackberries
1 warm low-carb tortilla with butter

LUNCH Bacon cheeseburger, "protein style"[1] (with tomato, onion, mustard, mayo, and pickle as desired)
1 pear

SNACK 1–2 ounces hard salami, 1 ounce hard cheese, 1 kiwi

DINNER Rotisserie or baked take-out chicken
½ cup zucchini sautéed in olive oil with ½ cup diced canned tomatoes and a sprinkling of Parmesan cheese
Green salad with choice of low-carb dressing
½ cup fresh or frozen blueberries with a dollop of whipped cream

Day 2

BREAKFAST 8 ounces plain yogurt mixed with any flavor of whey protein powder and 1 ounce sliced almonds
1 slice buttered low-carb toast and 1 tablespoon low-sugar jam

LUNCH Chef salad (with leftover rotisserie chicken, 1 cup raw veggies, boiled egg, and cheese) and choice of low-carb dressing
1 peach (or ½ cup no-sugar-added canned peach slices)

SNACK 2 ounces string cheese and 1 cup grapes

---

1. "Protein style" means wrapped in two large lettuce leaves instead of buns. Conversely, you could choose to have a low-carb burger bun and skip the pear or keep the bottom of a bun and eat ½ a pear. See how it works?

DINNER   Grilled or broiled steak
            ½ cup boiled beets dressed with butter, salt, and pepper
            ½ cup green beans
            1 sliced fresh peach (or ½ cup unsweetened frozen) with a
                dollop of whipped cream if desired

Day 3

BREAKFAST   Sausage and cheese omelet
            1½ cups fresh or frozen melon
            1 slice low-carb buttered toast and 2 teaspoons no-sugar
                jam

LUNCH   Tuna salad wrap (tuna salad in a low-carb tortilla with
                lettuce, tomato, onion, mayo, mustard, and pickles as
                desired)
            ½ small banana

SNACK   2–3 ounces leftover steak or deli meat, ½ small banana

DINNER   Grilled or broiled pork chops
            ½ cup raw cauliflower, broccoli, and bell peppers tossed
                with ranch dressing
            ½ cup green peas
            ½ cup cooked apples or applesauce

Over the next four days, you may either repeat these meal plans or
select from among your favorite transition meals (or come up with your
own using the Protein and Carbohydrate Servings Lists) and simply add
another small serving of carbohydrates to your breakfast. After you've
completed the full seven days, it will be time to reassess your status.
Pause a moment now to take stock before moving on. During this first
week in maintenance . . .

Has your weight increased?   Yes ☐ No ☐
Has your waist size increased?   Yes ☐ No ☐
Has your blood pressure gone up?   Yes ☐ No ☐
Are your rings or shoes tighter?   Yes ☐ No ☐
Are you experiencing heartburn?   Yes ☐ No ☐

If the following values were initially abnormal, you may also wish to
repeat these tests:

Has your blood sugar risen?   Yes ☐ No ☐
Have your triglycerides increased?   Yes ☐ No ☐

If you've answered yes to any question, you should go back to the transition level of carbohydrates and remain there for a few more weeks. That level may indeed be your limit. You may wish to attempt to go to the first step of maintenance again in the near future, or you may find that you are content to remain at the slightly lower transition carb level, and that's fine. You've already seen that you get to enjoy a wide variety of foods in transition, including lots of fruits and vegetables and even some slightly starchier foods. Don't forget that increased activity means higher carb tolerance for most people. If you'd like to eat slightly more carbs, crank up your physical output and you may be able to. Likewise, don't forget to crank the carbs back down if your physical activity decreases for some reason.

If you've answered no to all questions, you can advance to Week 2 for a slightly higher carb intake if you desire. Remember, you may stop increasing your carbs at any point where you feel comfortably satisfied with the amount you're eating and at any point where you are stable in weight and health. At a lower level of carbs, you'll be able to consume more calories from other sources such as lean protein and healthful fats to maintain weight.

Week 2

Day 1

BREAKFAST ¾–1 cup cottage cheese
(add sausage links for L, XL, or XXL protein servings)
1 cup fresh or frozen melon
1 slice buttered low-carb toast

LUNCH   Grilled chicken sandwich, "protein style" (with bacon, avocado, onion, tomato, mayo, mustard, and pickle as desired)
Green salad with raw veggies, tomato wedges, and choice of low-carb dressing
1 banana

SNACK   1–2 ounces hard salami, 1 ounce hard cheese, ½ cup grapes

DINNER   Grilled or broiled salmon or other firm-fleshed fish
Green salad with tomato wedges and choice of low-carb
dressing
10 fresh asparagus spears sautéed in olive oil and garlic (or
¾ cup canned asparagus)
1 slice low-carb garlic toast (low-carb toasted bread,
butter, and garlic powder)
1 black fig, split, topped with 1 teaspoon soft blue cheese,
broiled

Day 2

BREAKFAST   Fruit power smoothie (4 ounces plain yogurt, ½ cup water,
1 cup frozen berries, strawberry protein powder, and
1 packet Splenda)

LUNCH   Grilled salmon and cheese patty melt sandwich (2 slices
buttered low-carb bread, leftover salmon, and 1 or 2
cheese slices, grilled)
Green salad, 1 cup raw broccoli, cauliflower, and red peppers tossed with choice of low-carb dressing

SNACK   2 to 4 deviled (or hardboiled) egg halves and ½ cup grapes

DINNER   Roasted chicken
½ cup green peas
½ cup summer squash, buttered
Salad greens with choice of dressing
½ cup fresh or frozen raspberries with a dollop of whipped
cream if desired

Day 3

BREAKFAST   Eggs any style
Breakfast steak, broiled or grilled
1 cup fresh or frozen melon
2 warm low-carb tortillas, buttered and spread with
2 teaspoons low-carb jam

LUNCH   Roasted chicken wrap (chicken in a warmed low-carb
tortilla with fresh spinach, tomato, onion, avocado,
mayo, mustard, and pickle as desired)

Celery and 5 or 6 carrot sticks with good low-carb ranch or blue cheese dressing

1 orange

SNACK   1–2 ounces dry roasted mixed nuts and 1 tangerine

DINNER   Grilled or broiled fish (salmon, halibut, swordfish, or tuna)

1 cup spaghetti squash, buttered and topped with ¼ cup marinara sauce

Salad greens with good olive oil dressing

1 slice low-carb garlic toast (low-carb toasted bread, butter, and garlic powder)

½ cup commercial low-carb ice cream (watch those sugar alcohols!)

Over the next four days you may either repeat these meal plans or select from among your favorite transition meals (or come up with your own using the Protein and Carbohydrate Servings Lists) and simply add another small serving of carbohydrates to your breakfast and lunch. After you've completed the full seven days, it will be time to reassess your status. Pause a moment at that point to take stock before moving on. During this second week in maintenance . . .

Has your weight increased?	Yes ☐ No ☐
Has your waist size increased?	Yes ☐ No ☐
Has your blood pressure crept up?	Yes ☐ No ☐
Are your rings or shoes tighter?	Yes ☐ No ☐
Are you experiencing heartburn?	Yes ☐ No ☐

If these values were initially elevated, you may wish to repeat these lab tests:

Has your blood sugar risen?	Yes ☐ No ☐
Have your triglycerides increased?	Yes ☐ No ☐

If you've answered yes to any question, you should go back to the maintenance Week 1 level of carbohydrates and remain there. That level may indeed be your limit. You may wish to attempt to increase to the second step of maintenance again in the near future, or you might find that you're content to remain where you are, and that's fine. You've already seen that you get to enjoy a wide variety of foods at that level, including lots of fruits and vegetables and even some slightly starchier foods. Don't forget that increased activity means higher carb tolerance for most people. If you'd like to eat slightly more carbs, crank up your physical output and you may be able to. Likewise, don't forget the crank the carbs back down if your physical activity declines for some reason.

If you've answered no to all questions, then you can advance to maintenance Week 3 for a slightly higher carb intake if you desire. Remember, you may stop increasing your carbs at any point where you feel comfortably satisfied with the amount you're eating and at any point where you are stable in weight and health. At a lower level of carbs, you'll be able to consume more calories from other sources such as lean protein and healthy fats to maintain weight.

Week 3

Day 1

BREAKFAST   2 slices low-carb French toast (2 slices low-carb bread
             dipped in 1 egg beaten with ¼ cup half and half and a
             dash of nutmeg and fried in butter until crisp and golden)
          ¼ cup commercial low-carb syrup
          Sausage links
          ½ cup fresh or frozen berries

LUNCH   Grilled chicken sandwich, "protein style"[2]
          Garden salad (greens with tomatoes, raw broccoli, cauli-
             flower, carrots, mushrooms, and choice of low-carb
             dressing)
          1 pear

SNACK   1–2 ounces hard salami, 1 ounce hard cheese, 4 to 6 Blue
          Diamond Nut Thin crackers, mustard

DINNER   Grilled lamb burger patties (or hamburger)
          1 fresh tomato, wedged, plus 2 ounces fresh mozzarella,
             cubed, sprinkled with fresh chopped basil and salt and

2. Remember, you could choose to have half a bun and half a pear or the whole bun and no pear at all. You can spend your carbs however you like, but you'll get more nutritional bang for your buck with the juicy piece of fruit than with two pieces of starch.

pepper, and drizzled with olive oil and a bit of balsamic vinegar

¾ cup buttered cooked carrots

1 peach, sliced and topped with a dollop of whipped cream if desired

Day 2

BREAKFAST   Scrambled eggs and veggies (sauté ½ cup spinach and diced tomato, 1 tablespoon each bell peppers, onion, and mushroom in butter until soft, add beaten eggs, and cook until set) topped with 1 dollop each of salsa and sour cream

1 low-carb tortilla, warm, buttered

1 or 2 sausage links (extra links for XL and XXL protein servings)

1 tangerine

LUNCH   Lamb burger wrap (leftover lamb burger wrapped in a warm low-carb tortilla with lettuce, tomato, onion, and mayo, or minted yogurt dressing on page 25)

Spinach salad (with fresh mushrooms, chopped hardboiled egg, and crumbled bacon) with good olive oil vinaigrette

1 peach

SNACK   2 ounces string cheese and 1 cup grapes

DINNER   Baby-back ribs with ¼ cup low-carb commercial BBQ sauce

1 cup no-sugar-added coleslaw (½ cup commercial slaw)

½ cup green beans

½ cup no-sugar-added cooked apples or applesauce

Day 3

BREAKFAST   Fruit power smoothie (blend 4 ounces plain yogurt, ½ cup water, 1 cup frozen berries, strawberry protein powder, and 1 packet Splenda)

Crisp bacon

LUNCH   Chicken salad–stuffed tomato (Slice a large tomato into wedges, cutting almost through, leaving stem end intact. Spread the wedges to form a "blossom," salt lightly, drizzle with olive oil vinaigrette, and fill with chicken salad.)

½ avocado, sliced

6 to 8 Blue Diamond Nut Thin crackers with butter (or ½ small roll)

1 cup fresh or frozen strawberries with a dollop of whipped cream

SNACK 1–2 ounces dry roasted mixed nuts and ½ tangerine

DINNER Pot roast (with onion, bell pepper, cauliflower, zucchini, and carrots)[3]

1 slice low-carb garlic toast (1 slice toasted low-carb bread, buttered, and sprinkled with garlic powder)

Green salad with choice of low-carb dressing

½ tangerine

Over the next four days, you may either repeat these meal plans or select from among your favorite transition meals (or come up with your own using the Protein and Carbohydrate Servings Lists) and simply add one small serving of carbohydrate to your breakfast, lunch, and dinner. After you've completed the full seven days, it will be time to reassess your status. Pause a moment now to take stock before moving on. During this third week in maintenance . . .

Has your weight increased?	Yes ☐	No ☐
Has your waist size increased?	Yes ☐	No ☐
Has your blood pressure gone up?	Yes ☐	No ☐
Are your rings or shoes tighter?	Yes ☐	No ☐
Are you experiencing heartburn?	Yes ☐	No ☐

If these values were initially elevated, you may wish to repeat these lab tests:

Has your blood sugar risen?	Yes ☐	No ☐
Have your triglycerides increased?	Yes ☐	No ☐

If you've answered yes to any question, you should go back to the maintenance Week 2 level of carbohydrates and remain there. That level

3. Use your favorite pot roast recipe, omitting the potatoes or the flour it may contain, and substituting an equivalent amount of cauliflower and zucchini or yellow squash. Plan on about ½ small onion, ½ carrot, ½ bell pepper, and ½ zucchini per serving. You can thicken with 1–2 teaspoons of guar gum or xantham gum or Thickenthin notStarch, a commercial low-carb thickener for sauces, available at many online and low-carb specialty stores.

may indeed be your limit. You may wish to attempt to increase to the third step of maintenance again in the near future, or you might find that you are content to remain where you are, and that's fine. You've already seen that you get to enjoy a wide variety of foods at that level, including lots of fruits and vegetables and even some slightly starchier foods. Don't forget that increased activity means higher carb tolerance for most people. If you'd like to eat slightly more carbs, crank up your physical output and you may be able to. Likewise, don't forget to crank the carbs back down if your physical activity declines for some reason.

If you've answered no to all questions, then you can advance to Week 4 for a slightly higher carb intake if you desire. Remember, you may stop increasing your carbs at any point where you feel comfortably satisfied with the amount you're eating and at any point where you are stable in weight and health. At a lower level of carbs you'll be able to consume more calories from other sources such as lean protein and healthful fats to maintain weight.

Week 4

Day 1

BREAKFAST   Yogurt and berries (8 ounces plain yogurt, ½ cup mixed fresh or frozen berries, and 1 packet Splenda)
Sausage links

LUNCH   Bacon cheeseburger, "protein style" (with tomato, onion, avocado, pickle, mayo, and mustard as desired)
Garden salad (greens with raw broccoli, cauliflower, carrots, mushrooms) and ranch or blue cheese dressing
4 or 5 Blue Diamond Nut Thin crackers with butter
1 peach

SNACK   6 Blue Diamond Nut Thin crackers with 2 tablespoons almond butter or low-sugar peanut butter and ½ cup grapes

DINNER   Baked or rotisserie chicken
½ cup beets (baked or boiled, fresh) with butter
½ cup cooked carrots, buttered
½ cup green peas

Green salad with tomato wedges and good low-carb
dressing

½ cup fresh blueberries with a dollop of whipped cream

Day 2

BREAKFAST   Eggs any style
Crisp bacon
2 slices low-carb toast with butter and low-carb jam
½ banana

LUNCH   Roast chicken wrap (leftover chicken in a warm low-carb
tortilla, with fresh spinach leaves, tomatoes, fresh mozzarella slices, fresh basil leaves, and kalamata or black
olives, drizzled with olive oil and a splash of balsamic
vinegar)
1 orange

SNACK   1–2 ounces hard salami, 1–2 ounces cheddar cheese,
1 apple

DINNER   Roasted pork
½ cup black-eyed peas
2 cups raw broccoli, cauliflower, and bell peppers tossed
with olive oil and vinegar or buttermilk ranch dressing,
topped with 1 ounce toasted sliced almonds
1 slice low-carb garlic toast (toasted low-carb bread, butter, and garlic powder)
½ cup cooked no-sugar-added apples or applesauce

Day 3

BREAKFAST   Poached eggs, Canadian bacon
2 slices low-carb toast, buttered
Asparagus, steamed, with hollandaise if desired
1 cup fresh or frozen melon

LUNCH   BBQ pork wrap (leftover roast pork reheated with
1 tablespoon minced onion, 1–2 ounces low-carb
barbecue sauce, wrapped in a warm low-carb tortilla,
with dill pickles or pickled peppers)
½ cup no-sugar-added coleslaw
1 apple

SNACK   1–2 ounces deli turkey or chicken, 1 ounce string cheese,
               1 pear

DINNER   Grilled or broiled steak
               Sautéed or creamed spinach
               Fresh tomato salad (wedges of red and/or yellow tomatoes,
                   slivers of sweet onion, and capers dressed with good
                   olive oil vinaigrette)
               ¼ medium baked potato with skin (medium-sized, with but-
                   ter, sour cream, chives, and bacon crumbles as desired)[4]

Over the next four days, you may either repeat these meal plans or select from among your favorite transition meals (or come up with your own using the Protein and Carbohydrate Servings Lists) and simply add one small serving of carbohydrate to your breakfast, lunch, dinner, and snack. After you've completed the full seven days, it will be time to reassess your status. Pause a moment now to take stock before moving on. During this fourth week in maintenance . . .

Has your weight increased?   Yes ☐ No ☐
Has your waist size increased?   Yes ☐ No ☐
Has your blood pressure crept up?   Yes ☐ No ☐
Are your rings or shoes tighter?   Yes ☐ No ☐
Are you experiencing heartburn?   Yes ☐ No ☐

If these values were initially elevated, you may wish to repeat these lab tests:

Has your blood sugar risen?   Yes ☐ No ☐
Have your triglycerides increased?   Yes ☐ No ☐

If you've answered yes to any question, you should back up to the maintenance Week 3 level of carbohydrates and remain there. That level may indeed be your limit. You may wish to attempt to increase to the fourth step of maintenance again in the near future, or you might find

---

4. Potatoes are like sugar; they quickly run your blood sugar up. Treat them with caution. Keep the size small to medium and don't let ¼ become ½ or more! Or do as we do; scrape most of the flesh from inside the potato and discard it, dress the empty skin with all the fix-ings, and enjoy. You could enjoy 2–3 cups of summer squash or any large serving of a veggie or a fruit instead of ¼ baked potato; which do you prefer? As always, it's your call.

that you are content to remain where you are, and that's fine. You've already seen the tremendous amount and the wide variety of foods you can enjoy at that level, including more fruits and vegetables than you may ever have eaten before and respectable portions of some slightly starchier foods as well. Don't forget that increased activity means higher carb tolerance for most people. If you'd like to eat slightly more carbs, crank up your physical output and you may be able to. Likewise, don't forget to crank the carbs back down if your physical activity declines for some reason.

If you answered no to all questions, you are quite tolerant of a fairly high intake of good carbohydrates. There is no reason for you to continue to increase your intake unless you're still losing weight—an unlikely scenario unless your activity level is quite high for some reason, such as when participating in or training for major athletic competitions. If so, then continue to add small servings of fruits, vegetables, and bread or cereal grains to your meals until you finally reach your limit. And don't forget the law of intake and output: activity up, carbs up; activity down, carbs down.

Now that you've found your maintenance balance point, your job is to keep your commitment. In the next chapter, we'll give you some strategies for doing that.

CHAPTER 4

Maintenance: The Balancing Act

Corrective dieting is a sort of artificial environment. Many people view it as a set of nutritional handcuffs worn for a specific period of time to achieve a specific goal, often for a specific special event: a wedding, a reunion, or a major social occasion. And that's fine. Whatever motivates you to take control of your health, we're all for it. But maintenance is a lifelong program, and it can't be artificial. Your maintenance strategy has to be real and in sync with life as you live it, which could mean fitting your maintenance to your life or the reverse, making some deep reforms in your thinking. More often, it turns out to be a combination of the two.

Over the years, our patients have shown us a variety of ways to maintain the balance. Some opt for a careful control of their carbohydrate intake at their maintenance level at each meal and each snack, every day, throughout the year. These people recognize in themselves a need for tight control and feel that they'll operate better over the long haul working within a very defined carb allotment. This method seems to work well for people who are either very carb sensitive or who feel they might go on a carb bender if they relax their control.

Some of our patients opt for a relatively free weekend plan. These maintainers choose to follow their transition or even corrective level diet during the week and then eat pretty much whatever they want on the weekend. In our experience, this method, though it has its appeal in a regular reward of semi-indulgence, will only work for rather active, never-very-carb-sensitive people. And it demands that you climb back aboard the low-carb express every Monday morning.

In the past, a number of our patients approached maintenance in a slightly different way: instead of eating as many carbohydrates as their metabolism would allow each day in maintenance, they opted to control their carbohydrates a little more strictly, keeping to a transition level intake and eating more calories in protein and good fats. Then, once a month, they picked a day to enjoy the biggest, gooey-est, most delicious dessert they could find. They called themselves the "Dessert of the Month Club."

While their method worked well for them, it might not be so effective for others. Certainly, it was beneficial psychologically to plan for and enjoy the occasional high-carb fling, or, as we long ago termed it, a dietary vacation, but this eating pattern does have a metabolic impact. For most people, it might mean a bit of a metabolic hangover—a pound or two of fluid retention and tight rings for a day or two, but easily recoverable with a couple of days of Low-Carb Boot Camp (see "7-Day Low-Carb Boot Camp" later in this chapter). Other people, however, are sensitive enough to sugar that partaking in such an indulgence would send them spiraling out of control.

Know yourself. If you know that one gooey dessert would lead to two or three or more, don't attempt a maintenance lifestyle that will set you up to fail. And don't be fooled into believing that because you weigh less or have lowered your blood pressure, you've somehow received a metabolism transplant. If your inherent tendency toward insulin resistance resulted in weight gain or elevated blood pressure or higher lab values in the past, that tendency remains.

As you enter this period of what ideally will be lifelong maintenance, you'll want to examine the aspects of your daily life that have the potential to interfere with your goal of maintaining your health and/or weight. Can you pinpoint trouble spots, habitual activities, or even friends or associates (diet saboteurs) who have in the past exerted a negative pull on your good intentions? If you can, you're in a good position to devise a positive plan of counteraction.

For instance, suppose you have developed a daily habit of stopping by the coffee bar on the way to work for an extra-large six-pump white chocolate mocha—a more-than-600-calorie proposition with heaven knows how many grams of carbs. Unless your walk to work takes several hours at a pretty high intensity, you won't work off this daily fix, and, ultimately, you'll probably begin to gain weight or see your blood values climb again. You could avoid this maintenance destroyer by (1) changing your route and walking another way that doesn't take you past the coffee bar; (2) keeping your same route, still dropping into the coffee bar, but choosing a large hot tea or a decaf Americano; or (3) dropping in for a more reasonably sized white chocolate mocha every other Tuesday. Only you can say which method would work best for you.

More than anything else, successful maintenance is a balancing act, a series of small daily sacrifices and a few triumphs punctuated by the occasional slide or slip, and afterward, a recovery of equilibrium. That balancing-act mind-set will hold you in good stead; you'll be able to maintain as long as you keep a clear eye on your status by regular monitoring. Set upper limits for your weight and lab numbers; a reasonable limit might be no greater than a 10-pound increase in weight and a sustained increase (meaning two readings in a row pushing up against or mildly outside the normal range limit for that test) in any critical lab value such as blood sugar, cholesterol, triglycerides, insulin, or blood pressure.

Monitoring Your Maintenance

How often should you monitor your status? It's really up to you and what works best in your particular case. Through the years, we've witnessed the maintenance journeys of thousands of patients and heard from thousands of readers who want to share their stories with us. From them, we've learned that there are probably as many ways to approach maintenance as there are people trying to maintain. What works for one person may not work for another, so we're providing you with some of the most popular methods and, in them, we trust that you'll find one suitable to your own lifestyle.

We recall a patient who maintained his weight for many years by weighing daily. If his weight was up that day, he ate a Boot Camp menu; if it was stable or down, he ate his maintenance level menu. That's keeping a pretty tight rein on things, but it worked well for him. Notice the word *him*. Daily weighing is not necessarily as good an option for women, since women's weight can be influenced strongly by the fluid retention that comes naturally with hormonal cycles, and a transient increase may not indicate actual fat regain. However, this method could work to the benefit even of women, chiefly because during times of hormonal fluid retention, sticking to a lower-carb diet will help to reduce the effects of retention. It's not a bad maintenance strategy to spend a day or two in Low-Carb Boot Camp each month to help offset the cyclic fluid gain.

More often, our patients and readers report that they continue to weigh weekly, setting an upper limit for weight regain of 5 pounds. Once they reach that limit, they return to Low-Carb Boot Camp until their weight falls back to their maintenance baseline. Then they ease back through a week of transition and into maintenance.

Some people never weigh themselves—not a bad idea, since weight is really quite a crude measure of health and fitness. Some rely on following measurements of their body composition (body fat percentage) and others rely on size—do their jeans fit comfortably? Are their waistbands pinching? Have they quit wearing certain items in their closet because they're tight? For these folks, the minute their favorite jeans start to feel snug, it's back to Low-Carb Boot Camp until they're comfortable again. Whatever frequency of weight monitoring or size monitoring you choose, be sure to keep a running record in the Progress Chart in your journal.

Finally, for people who are concerned about maintaining control of their health issues, regular monitoring (by themselves or their physicians) is the key to success. It's a simple matter to determine whether symptoms of reflux or sleep apnea have returned. And it's easy to check your blood pressure or blood sugar at home. But it requires your doctor's cooperation to monitor changes in your cholesterol, triglycerides, uric acid, or inflammatory markers. In holding the line on health maintenance, your best course of action is to set regular annual (or even better, if possible, semiannual) appointments for health screening. Keep a careful record of your readings in the Progress Chart in your journal. At the first sign of elevated readings, you should go back to Boot Camp, regain control, and then gently ease back into your maintenance lifestyle.

We encourage you to approach the idea of maintenance with the same zeal and excitement that you brought to rehabilitating your health and body at the outset of your diet. Dedicate yourself to maintaining your weight and your health for the rest of your life, and you will. In this chapter, you'll learn some of the techniques that have helped our patients keep their commitment to maintenance throughout the years. We are sure they'll help you, too.

The Law of Intake and Output, or How to Balance on Three Legs

Research has shown that as many as 75 percent of us have a tendency to develop insulin resistance to a greater or lesser degree if we overeat carbohydrates. That leaves 25 percent of people who can eat almost anything and suffer no apparent health or weight consequences; we long ago termed these individuals the metabolically gifted and talented, and they have no need of this book.

Because the tendency toward insulin resistance and all the disorders it can spawn appears to be inherited, whether you fall into the 75 percent or the 25 percent is pretty much the genetic luck of the draw. Those of us in the 75 percent know who we are—we're the ones who have to work at not gaining weight; have a hard time losing weight; struggle to keep it off; suffer from or have a family history of metabolic disorders such as high blood pressure, diabetes, and heart disease; and respond very well to a low-carb diet.

But diet is only part of the equation. Weight control over the long haul is like a three-legged stool: one leg is carb intake, one leg is calorie intake, and one leg is calorie output. As long as all three legs are stable, the stool will balance, but if one of them breaks, the stool will fall. So it is with the balance you'll find in maintenance. Even after you've advanced through to your carbohydrate maximum, your game plan must remain flexible.

Your tolerance of carbohydrates is to some extent dependent on your level of activity, what you can think of as your physical output. The more active you are, the more carbs you will likely tolerate. If your level of activity changes, you'll need to adjust your carb intake to match your reduced physical output. We call it the Law of Intake and Output, and it's worth remembering because, like most laws, it's tough to get around, and obeying it will usually keep you out of trouble.

It works like this: say your habit is to play tennis twice a week with a friend, but you sprain your ankle and can't play. You'll need to reduce your carbohydrate intake or your calorie intake or both to match your decrease in activity, or you'll probably pick up a few pounds—that is, unless you can find some other activity to do with your bum ankle that will burn an equal number of calories. Otherwise, it's dietary adjustment time. Of the two options, we'd recommend cutting the carb intake and not the calories, because if you're injured, the nutrient your body will need most to heal is protein, not carb. You might get by just moving back to the transition carb level, but you may even have to return to the corrective level of intake for a few weeks to maintain your weight while you rehabilitate your injury. Once you're healed and ready to resume a more active life, you can add those carbs back into your diet. Failure to heed this law has packed pounds on many an injured athlete—both the weekend variety and the professional one. Remember, it's activity up, carbs up; activity down, carbs down. More specifically, we should say: activity up, carbs *can* go up; activity down, carbs *better* go down or weight *will* go up!

Warren's Tale

Warren came to our clinic about ten years ago at a weight of nearly 350 pounds. Always a big guy—he was a football lineman in his younger years—he was accustomed to unrestrained eating of heaping portions at every meal; he became a poster child for the All-American high-everything diet: high-fat, high-carb, high-protein, and high-calorie. The inactivity of adulthood and his family history caught up with him in his 30s, and he watched helplessly as his weight ballooned, his waistline expanded, and his health declined. By the time he came to see us, he was taking two medications for blood pressure and one for cholesterol, while chomping antacid tablets around the clock. For more than a year, he had exercised regularly, cut his fat intake to the bone, and staved off hunger between pasta dinners with carrot sticks and fat-free bagels. That strategy had gotten him almost zero results, except that now his family doctor felt he needed a fourth medication to control his blood sugar. At his wits' end, he decided to try the low-carb approach.

Warren approached his new regimen with fervor, able to stick closely to the plan since, as he put it, "at least I get something decent to eat on it." The combination of a sensible low-carb corrective diet and his previous exercise regimen paid off; in just a little over six months, he lost more than 100 pounds and was able to discontinue two of his three medications. He told us that he felt as if a whole new life had opened up for him: he bought new clothes, changed jobs, and fell in love with a woman he met while traveling in Europe.

Then, about six months into his maintenance, life threw him a curveball. His fiancée, whom he was expecting to arrive in the States within days, called to say that she couldn't do it. She wasn't coming; the wedding was off. When he came to the clinic that week and told us what had happened, we listened and then asked the obvious: so what did you do? He responded, "I ate two entire tubes of raw chocolate chip cookie dough in front of the TV." We talked about that and about alternative (and less self-destructive) coping strategies: going for a good hard workout at the gym, taking a long walk, going with friends to a game or a movie, reading an engrossing book, or talking with a friend, a counselor, or a pastor. We reminded Warren that focusing on something that will make a positive impact in his life—volunteering in the community, mowing the lawn, raking the leaves, trimming the hedges, washing the windows, or cleaning out the garage, the attic, the storage room, or the closet—can be therapeutic. Choosing to become involved in these kinds of activities has a twofold benefit: it serves to distract you from unhappy thoughts and gives you a feeling of accomplishment and control, because the result of the effort is something you can feel good about.

Warren took our suggestions to heart, and before long he was feeling better about his life again. Although still nursing his broken heart, he had no more run-ins with the cookie dough. Then disaster struck again. One day at the gym, he ruptured his biceps tendon, a severe injury that required surgery and put his right arm in a cast from fingertips to shoulder for a couple of months. While he appeared to have weathered the first blow, we feared that this second one—both emotional and physical—could derail his maintenance. We reminded him of the Law of Intake and Output and of the need to take up some other form of exercise, to cut his intake of either carbs or calories, or both. He assured us that he understood and would try.

Warren was understandably depressed by these events, so we also suggested a mild antidepressant medication and a referral for counseling to help him work through the depression, but he declined. He felt that he could do it on his own; we weren't as convinced. And sure enough, week by week, his weight climbed until he had regained almost half of what he'd lost. Finally, we persuaded him to let us help, and with counseling and medication (and finally the full healing of his injury), he was able to get his weight back down and his maintenance back on track.

7-Day Low-Carb Boot Camp

Warren's story isn't especially unusual. In our experience with thousands of overweight patients during two decades of clinical practice, we'd say it's less the exception than the rule. One of the chief contributors to the all-too-common cycle of weight loss and regain is being emotionally unprepared for the curveballs that life throws us. And since life's got more curves than a major league bullpen, it behooves us all—if we hope to win the maintenance game—to have a plan in place.

We designed the Low-Carb Boot Camp week as the nutritional centerpiece of your recovery plan. Because it's nearly impossible to please all palates, you may encounter a meal that contains something you can't or won't eat. Should that arise, you may do a little horse trading. All meals are interchangeable—that is, you may swap any breakfast for another breakfast, any lunch for another lunch, any dinner for another dinner, or any snack for another snack. You may also substitute any protein food (meat, fish, poultry, or game) for something else from your Protein Servings Lists for the meat part of any meal—say, chicken for steak, pork chops for lamb chops, or salmon for hamburger. Do not, however, substitute the fruits and the veggies, since they've been pretty carefully matched to keep you on a very controlled carb level for the recovery week. A few other rules apply in Boot Camp as well:

1. No alcohol, not so much as a light beer or a glass of wine. It's only for a week; you can do it! And it's important to help get your fat burning back on track by giving your liver a breather for a week.

2. No between-meal snacking except for the single specified snack, which you should eat at a time that will interrupt your longest stretch without food. For some people, that could be midmorning; for others, late afternoon. It's okay not to have the snack at all if you feel satisfied by just your three meals.

3. No more than two cups of caffeinated coffee a day, sweetened if you like with Splenda or stevia and lightened with a little heavy cream or half and half. No lattes or mochas. Again, you're limiting caffeine to give your liver a breather. You can choose to go fully decaf if you like, but if you're used to your coffee, you may develop a caffeine-withdrawal headache.

4. Acceptable beverages include water, mineral water, decaf coffee or tea, or herbal tea.

5. Acceptable dressings are those low in carbs—oil-based or cream-based dressings such as ranch, blue cheese, olive oil vinaigrette, plain oil and vinegar, or lemon juice—in a nutshell, dressings that don't contain more than a couple of grams of carbs per serving.

6. Be absolutely certain to supplement with magnesium and potassium each day. Shifting abruptly to a very-low-carb diet causes a dramatic drop in insulin and blood sugar that will cause a rapid release of excess retained body fluid and an increase in urine production. With this will come a loss of potassium and magnesium that can lead to a feeling of fatigue or muscle cramps. For this reason, these two nutrients require active replacement during this week. For most people, we'd recommend 3 or 4 over-the-counter tablets, most of which contain about 99 mg of magnesium and 99 mg of potassium each. You should be able to locate an acceptable combination magnesium/potassium product at any health food store, vitamin shop, or online. If you have difficulty finding one, check our Web site at www.proteinpower.com. (If you currently take medication for fluid or blood pressure, check with your pharmacist to be sure your medication does not promote potassium retention before you supplement with extra potassium.) It's really important that you supplement during Boot Camp.

Boot Camp Meals

Day 1

BREAKFAST   Eggs any style
Crisp bacon
½ cup fresh strawberries

LUNCH   Grilled hamburger patty(s) with cheese
1–2 cups salad greens with ½ fresh tomato and choice of
low-carb dressing

SNACK   1–2 ounces raw or dry roasted almonds

DINNER   Herbed grilled chicken (brush chicken with melted butter;
sprinkle on rosemary, oregano, basil, garlic, salt and
pepper; and grill or roast)
½ cup broccoli, steamed and dressed with olive oil, salt,
and pepper
1–2 cups salad greens with ½ fresh tomato and choice of
low-carb dressing

Day 2

BREAKFAST   Hi-Protein Shake (blend ¾ cup water, ¼ cup half and
half, any flavor protein powder, Splenda to sweeten, and
ice to thicken if desired)

LUNCH   Grilled chicken wrap (leftover grilled chicken wrapped in
a low-carb tortilla, with raw spinach, onion, tomato,
mayo, mustard, and pickle as desired)
⅓ cup grapes

SNACK   1 ounce salami, 1 ounce cheese, ½ fresh orange

DINNER   Grilled lamb chops (rub with olive oil, chopped basil,
oregano, mint, garlic, salt, and pepper)
½ cup eggplant sautéed in olive oil and garlic
1–2 cups salad greens with choice of low-carb dressing

Day 3

BREAKFAST   Ham and cheese omelet
½ cup strawberries, fresh or frozen unsweetened
1 slice buttered low-carb toast (no more than 6 effective
grams of carb)

LUNCH   Lamb chef salad (cubed leftover lamb, 1–2 cups salad
greens, 1 ounce feta cheese, 4 or 5 kalamata olives,
1 hard-cooked egg, 1 cup raw broccoli and cauliflower,
½ fresh tomato) with low-carb dressing of choice

SNACK   1 ounce peanuts and ½ fresh orange

DINNER   Baked, broiled, or grilled ocean fish (salmon, tilapia, snapper, mahi mahi, or halibut)

5 or 6 spears asparagus, sautéed or roasted (or ½ cup canned)

1–2 cups salad greens

½ cup raspberries (fresh or frozen) with a dollop of whipped cream

Day 4

BREAKFAST Strawberry protein smoothie (1 cup water, ½ cup frozen strawberries, strawberry low-carb protein powder)

LUNCH   Fish tacos (leftover fish wrapped in a warm low-carb tortilla, dressed with ¼ cup shredded green cabbage, ½ tomato, diced, and mayo spiked with a squeeze of lime juice and a pinch of cumin and chili powder)

SNACK   ½ fresh orange and 1 ounce string cheese

DINNER   Grilled or broiled steak

1 cup raw broccoli, cauliflower, and red bell pepper tossed with 1 ounce buttermilk ranch or blue cheese dressing

⅓ cup cooked winter squash (acorn, butternut, or hubbard) topped with a pat of butter and a sprinkle of salt, pepper, and cinnamon

Day 5

BREAKFAST Eggs any style

Sausage patties

Berry slush (½ cup unsweetened frozen mixed berries, ½ cup water, and 1 packet Splenda or stevia)

LUNCH   Shrimp salad in avocado (½ avocado filled with tiny canned shrimp, dressed with a mixture of 1 tablespoon mayo, 1 tablespoon low-carb catsup, a squeeze of lemon juice, salt, and pepper) on a bed of mixed lettuces

1 small low-carb tortilla, warmed and buttered

SNACK   1 cup raw broccoli, cauliflower, and carrots with 2 ounces ranch dressing

DINNER   Hamburger patty(s)

½ cup mushrooms, sautéed in olive oil and garlic
1–2 cups salad greens and ½ tomato with choice of low-
carb dressing

Day 6

BREAKFAST New York breakfast wrap (eggs, scrambled with lox[1] and
1 ounce cream cheese, wrapped in a warm small low-
carb tortilla)
½ fresh tomato, sliced

LUNCH Open-faced cheeseburger (leftover patty[s] on a slice of
low-carb bread, topped with 1 ounce melted cheese)
1 cup salad greens with choice of low-carb dressing

SNACK ½ tangerine and 1 ounce roasted almonds

DINNER Grilled or broiled kielbasa or Polish sausage
½ cup sauerkraut
1 cup raw broccoli, cauliflower, and red bell pepper tossed
with olive oil vinaigrette

Day 7

BREAKFAST Protein berry shake (½ cup unsweetened frozen mixed
berries, ¼ cup half and half, 1 cup water, and vanilla
low-carb protein powder)

LUNCH Open-faced sausage sandwich (1 slice low-carb bread,
leftover grilled sausage, pickle, mustard, lettuce leaves,
tomato, and onion slices as desired)
⅓ cup grapes

SNACK ⅓ cup grapes and 1–2 ounces hard cheese

DINNER Roast beef
½ cup green beans
½ cup steamed broccoli and cauliflower, topped with
1 ounce melted cheese

When you've really fallen off the wagon or your weight has crept up
to your preset upper limit, you'll need to spend the full week in Boot

---

1. Substitute a different breakfast protein if you prefer.

Camp. Once you've completed your time there, you should return to the transition level for a week or so and then move back into maintenance. It's also fine to spend a day or two in Boot Camp, as discussed in this chapter, to recover from a one-time carb splurge or to shed some fluid you've retained from hormone cycles. In that event, you can just spend a day or two in Boot Camp and then go right back onto maintenance.

Danger: Curves Ahead

Chief among the curves along life's road are what we call the Big 7 or the seven major life stresses. Here they are:

1. death of a loved one
2. divorce or separation
3. serious injury to self or a loved one
4. serious illness of self or a loved one
5. financial collapse
6. loss of employment
7 loss of a long-sought-after goal

Getting hit with one (or more) of the Big 7 can cause any of us to feel anxiety, depression, sleeplessness, and fear. But for many people, especially those who have struggled with their weight, these stresses can inspire the desire to eat. Just about all of us, at one time or another, have drawn comfort from food. From childhood tears dried with promises of ice cream and candy to teenage broken hearts soothed with chocolate chip cookies and milk, we've come to associate certain types of food with comfort and security. Traditional comfort foods—such as mashed potatoes and gravy, pancakes and syrup, macaroni and cheese, cookies, brownies, ice cream, chips, and candy—all share one common theme: they're stout doses of both carbohydrates and fat. And for a person with a tendency for insulin-related problems (and remember 75 percent of us have some degree of this tendency), these kinds of foods will easily upset our metabolic balance. That's not to say that the occasional serving of mashed potatoes will undo your maintenance, nor will the occasional stack of pancakes. The danger of these comforts, in our experience, lies more in your intent in eating them than in the insulin-elevating effect of the food itself.

Is that serving of macaroni and cheese a celebration or a reward, or it is solace? The distinction is an important one, because a celebratory indulgence is usually a one-time deal. Congratulations on your promotion, your acceptance to law school, or the sale of your book! It usually happens infrequently, you celebrate, and that's that. The use of food in an attempt to find solace from hurt or anxiety, however, is often repetitive; since the food just makes you feel good temporarily and doesn't really solve the problem, the cause of the anxiety or the hurt remains, and often the need to seek comfort from food continues with it.

Examine your own tendencies. Under emotional stress, do you reach for comfort in food? If so, this behavior will haunt you in maintenance unless you make a plan of action now to counter it. Among the most important of your defense strategies is simply recognizing that you indeed have a tendency to seek comfort in food under stress. Let's look at some alternatives.

1. Put distance between yourself and the food you typically turn to under stress. Go through your kitchen cupboards, refrigerator, or desk drawer and throw out your go-to foods. Do not repurchase them even if someone else in the house likes them. Limiting easy access to the foods that sorely tempt you at a time of stress may not always prevent a slip, but it will at least make it easier to resist the temptation.

2. Put distance between yourself and the place where you tend to eat when stressed. Try to pinpoint the time of day or the location that seems to be the trouble zone. If you find that you eat in front of the television in the evening, plan to get out of the house after a sensible dinner. Walk the dog, join an exercise group, attend a lecture, volunteer with a local charity, mentor a child, or take an art class. A shakeup in your normal routine will put you farther from the danger zone, and you may even meet a whole new array of interesting people.

3. Substitute another activity for eating. As we mentioned before, when you feel the desire to soothe stress with food, it's possible to redirect that impulse by involving yourself in some other project: gardening, sewing, painting, cleaning, organizing, woodworking, or any of a hundred other activities you might find interesting.

4. Substitute foods that are more metabolically neutral. For instance, if you tend to go for mac and cheese, try just having the cheese. If ice cream is your downfall, try having one of the low-carb varieties that's now on the market. While this option doesn't address the underlying tendency to eat under stress, at least these kinds of low-carb choices won't send your insulin back through the roof.

5. Seek professional help if symptoms of depression or anxiety persist. Don't wait, like Warren, until you've eaten yourself halfway back to where you started from before asking for help. There is no shame in becoming anxious or depressed when one of these major life stresses hits you broadside. Speak with your physician, your clergyman, or your local mental health services provider to obtain counseling, direction, and, if needed, medication to help you through an emotional rough patch.

The Big 7 certainly aren't the only emotional causes that unhinge weight and health maintenance. Smaller, chronic, day-to-day stresses can undermine your intentions too. To help you withstand those kinds of stress, think about this: no matter what the problem is, unless it's starvation, food won't solve it. It may take your mind off it and make you feel momentarily soothed, but it won't fix the problem. It could, however, threaten your maintenance. Let's look at how one man approached the stress in his life. It's the story of our friend Jack. We wrote about Jack years ago, we've related his story to our patients through the years, and we think his story will inspire you to stay committed to your goals in maintenance.

Discipline As an Art Form: Jack Strikes Back

About fifteen years ago, Jack, an old college friend, paid us a visit. He was driving through our part of the country with his wife, who was afflicted with AIDS, which she had contracted from a foreign blood transfusion several years earlier. Our friend—a petroleum engineer—lived in Houston, where he designed refineries for one of the major oil companies. In the late 1980s the petroleum industry had suffered a severe economic downturn, resulting in many layoffs, staff transfers, and consolidations (improbable as that scenario seems to us now in an era of

$50-a-barrel crude oil). By virtue of his ability and length of employment, Jack had been able to avoid most of the upheaval, but, unfortunately, it finally caught up with him. He was transferred from his department and put on leave of absence until his new position—one that he didn't want—was open. He took the several weeks available and spent them traveling with his wife to visit family and friends across the country, including us.

The last time we'd seen Jack, six or so years earlier, he had started to develop a little middle-aged spread, and we expected him to be heavier still. We were very surprised to open the door and find him looking trim and fit. Later at dinner at one of our favorite restaurants, one that specializes in fabulous dessert concoctions (we were planning a little dietary vacation in honor of their visit), we noticed that Jack ate a steak, a salad, and some vegetables and couldn't be persuaded even to nibble anything from the dessert tray. He had coffee while the rest of us plowed into some delicious gooey dessert that we later regretted having eaten. Knowing his predilection for sweets in the past (he lived on them in college), we asked him about the change. His response—the reasoned reaction of a very rational mind—caused us to change our thinking on the whole idea of eating.

"Guys, my life is in enormous turmoil. My wife is sick with a disease that I can't understand and can't do anything about." Remember, back in those early days of the AIDS epidemic, there were no treatments of any kind available. "My job is in jeopardy, and now I've been moved—against my will—to a position that I don't want and probably can't perform very well. I had no choice—it was either change or resign, and with Nancy's illness, I couldn't afford to be without insurance, so even my option to resign was taken away. I'm being bounced along by events over which I have no control whatsoever—I can't control this disease and I can't control what happens to me at work. In fact, I don't know how long I'll be in this new position or if I'll even be working beyond that. At this point, my diet, my weight, and my physical condition are a few of the only things left in my life that I *can* control—and I intend to control them. That's why I watch my diet and don't eat sweets."

Prompted by his eloquent, well-reasoned response, we began to think very seriously about this business of control over eating. Most people have the reverse of the problem that Jack had—they are in control of most aspects of their lives but feel completely out of control when it comes to their eating. In our years of medical practice, we've seen so many people who are professionals of one sort or another—executives, politicians, even career military officers—who overeat and are over-weight. These people hold demanding positions that require consider-able self-discipline and sacrifice. They don't hesitate to throw themselves fully into projects that entail monumental sacrifices of their time and energy; they are exacting people who demand near perfection in them-selves and others. Yet they seem unable to control their own eating, in great measure because they, unlike our friend Jack, don't look upon eat-ing as something that is subject to their control. But it is.

There are many circumstances over which we have no control what-soever. The weather, the economy, the actions of our coworkers, the mis-deeds of elected officials, the misbehavior of grown children—all these things and many like them we have little control over, yet we find our-selves worrying about them, considering all sorts of options to effect change in the behavior of other people or to modify affairs that we have no power to modify. We're not saying that we can't insulate ourselves from changes in the economy, inclement weather, actions of other peo-ple, and so on, because we can; we just can't change those things them-selves. We waste who knows how much time and emotional energy in trying to change situations we can't change; *yet we often refuse to change the situations over which we have complete control.*

You may not be able to control anything else, but you can control your eating. Sure, dieting requires some discipline and self-control, espe-cially in the beginning. Maintaining your dietary commitment to better health and fitness will require focus and determination for years to come. But you should regard your diet and your new slimmer, healthier body as you would anything else that needs effort to maintain. You wouldn't work diligently and sacrifice your time and energy to obtain a better job, only to slack off, loaf, and get fired after being hired. Why do it with your diet? When you were in school, you didn't stay up late with your nose in a book and sacrifice your weekends studying to do well on an exam, only to make a halfhearted effort and blow it. Why do it with your diet? If you have reached adulthood, gone to school, and main-tained a job, you have exercised discipline. You may feel that you have exercised more or less discipline than others, but you have exercised discipline nevertheless. And discipline, like any other skill, becomes more proficient with use. Use it.

If circumstances arise that burden you emotionally, don't bolt from your diet and seek comfort in food. Analyze the situation and determine whether you can do anything about it. If you can, take the appropriate action; if not, recognize the fact and try to focus your energies elsewhere. You will always have control of your diet. Don't relinquish it. To better learn how to flex your discipline muscles, we highly recommend an excellent book on the subject: *Take Effective Control of Your Life* by William Glasser, M.D. Even if you're living a problem-free life, this book will help you, and if, like our friend Jack, you find yourself beset by one or more of life's major stresses, you'll profit enormously from it.

Dr. Glasser says that there are four components to any behavior: the doing component, the feeling component, the thinking component, and the physiological component. Of the four, we have complete control only over the doing component. We have partial control over the thinking component, but over the other two, we have no control whatsoever. Since Dr. Glasser touches on diet only peripherally in his book, let's look for a moment at how these components and our control over them apply to eating—and to strategies for maintenance.

Suppose, for example, that you haven't eaten for a time and you see or smell food that appeals to you; you feel hungry—the feeling component. You can't help it that you feel hungry; it's beyond your control. Your mouth waters and your stomach growls; these are the physiologic components. You can't keep your salivary glands from working, and you can't do anything about the increasing activity of your stomach's glands and muscles. None of us can. We have no control over these physiological processes.

So you look at the food and smell the aroma, and you imagine how good it will taste—and voilà—there's the thinking component. As long as you're hungry and in the presence of this wonderful food, you'll probably think about eating it. Who wouldn't? You can force yourself to think about other things, but more than likely, your thoughts will drift back to the food, and you'll have to rein them in again. So we can partially control our thinking—some of us more effectively than others. But if you sit down and eat the food, that's the doing component, and this act you can completely control. You can eat or not as you please. Unlike the workings of our salivary glands or our feelings of hunger, we all have total, 100 percent control over whether we actually put the food into our mouths and chew.

The interesting thing is that although many of us allow the uncontrollable components of behavior to direct the controllable one, it can work in the reverse direction. If you take charge of the doing component, over which you have total control, the involuntary components will fall into step. When confronted with dietary temptation, if you walk away from the food and involve yourself in a different activity, unrelated to food or eating, slowly your feelings, physiology, and thinking will change and adapt themselves to your new activity. You will have controlled the behavior that was possible to control, and as a result, you'll indirectly take control of what you thought you couldn't. And each time you do this, your discipline muscles get a little bit stronger.

Handling the Holidays

Second only to the stresses of life in their power to unhinge the best maintenance intentions is that annual period of dietary temptation that begins with "Trick or treat!" and ends with "Happy New Year!" Joyous as the celebratory feasts of our religious and cultural heritage may be, for most people, the holiday season is stressful. Combine all the traveling, the shopping, the budgeting, and the kids home from school with cookies, candy, and egg nog, and before you know it, it's: Oh, my! What happened to my maintenance plan? The designated eat-fest in the last quarter of the year packs between 5 and 12 pounds on the average American frame. Here are some tips to help you avoid this annual maintenance pitfall.

Halloween

Rethink the giving of Halloween candy and sugary treats, mindful of their impact on yourself, your family, and the kids who come to the door.

1. Consider giving nonedible treats, such as small party favor toys, small boxes of crayons, or other novelty items.
2. Pass out small bags of peanuts, sunflower seeds, nuts, jerky, trail mix, or other lower-carb homemade treats. After all, the kids don't really *need* more candy, do they?

3. Buy candy you don't like. If you feel you must give candy treats, purchase the kind of candy you don't especially like or at least one you have less weakness for. If a whole bowlful of your favorite candy sits around that evening and on the days after the trick-or-treating, some of it will surely find its way into your mouth. Sometimes, a lot of it will. Don't set yourself up for needless temptation.

4. Don't buy candy too early. Granted, the stores start putting it out just after Labor Day, but resist the urge to buy it too soon. If it sits on your cupboard or pantry shelf, it will serve only as a temptation to eat it. And whenever you buy it, don't open it until just before you expect to hear that first bing-bong at your door.

5. Throw (or give) away all leftover treats the next day—unless, of course, you opted for a low-carb alternative. Although it goes against our nature to toss out perfectly edible food, bear in mind that sugar and high-fructose corn syrup are really not nutritious food. They're full of calories and carbs—empty ones.

The Holiday Feasts

In the weeks leading up to the seasonal food fest—which for most of us begins with Thanksgiving—commit yourself with an added measure of focus to follow your nutritional regimen. You may even want to pare your carb intake back to a transitional or even a corrective level in preparation for the added food that's sure to come.

1. Plan to limit your indulgence to the actual day of the feast; try not to let the holiday eating patterns extend from several days before to a week afterward.

2. If you plan to undertake a lot of holiday baking, wait as long as you reasonably can to do it. Goodies that sit around are an open invitation to start the celebration early. Immediately freeze anything that can be frozen, and if possible, save the preparation of foods that can't be frozen or sealed away out of sight to the last few days, thereby limiting your easy access to them. Try new lower-carb recipes for holiday goodies. You'll find dozens of recipes for pies, cakes, cookies, and candies in our *Low-Carb Comfort Food Cookbook*, as well as in many of the other fine low-carb recipe collections now available in bookstores, magazines, and online. You'll be

able to enjoy them with less risk to your maintenance commitment.

3. Consider modifying your traditional holiday meals. The meat, fish, or poultry portion of most holiday meals—the turkey at Thanksgiving, the Christmas goose or ham—doesn't pose a problem. It's the side dishes and the desserts that can undo you. Many carb-rich dishes can be deliciously replaced by lower-carb options. For instance, substitute butternut squash for yams, cauliflower or celery root puree for mashed potatoes, and fresh cranberry relish sweetened with Splenda for cranberry jellies and sugar-based sauces. Seek out good lower-carb recipes for some of your holiday favorites; again, you'll find many low-carb comforts, from dressings and rolls to delicious side dishes, in our *Low-Carb Comfort Food Cookbook* and others. Shaving a few or more carbs off every item in your holiday cornucopia can make the feast much easier on your waistline.

4. Start your holiday morning with a high-protein, carb-controlled breakfast—bacon and eggs, cottage cheese with fresh fruit, or even a protein shake—to keep your blood sugar stable and your hunger at bay. You'll be less likely to nibble at higher-carb feast foods.

5. Begin your holiday feast with a clear soup course. Filling your stomach with a cup or two of clear broth soup and waiting a few minutes before digging into the main feast will take the edge off your ravenous holiday hunger. You'll find that you'll be satisfied with smaller portions on your plate.

6. Serve plenty of fresh, raw veggies—broccoli, cauliflower, celery and carrot sticks, and green onions—to add color, fiber, variety, and crunch.

7. Try to match the amount of food you prepare to the number of people you're feeding, so that you will have few, if any, leftovers, particularly of foods in the high-carb category. We know that leftovers are part of the enjoyment of a holiday feast—who doesn't like a turkey, dressing, and cranberry relish sandwich the next day? (Okay, two out of three of our own sons don't, but that's a story for another day.) If you love to enjoy leftovers for a day or two, then make enough for that, but don't go overboard.

8. If you choose to keep your traditional menu and recipes, try cutting your normal portions of the dressing, potatoes, yams, rolls, and desserts in half. Enjoy the food and then wait a full fifteen minutes after finishing these smaller portions before you consider going for seconds. You may be surprised to find that your satiety center has kicked in and you really don't feel hungry.

9. Consider starting new traditions. Volunteer to serve meals at a community kitchen on Thanksgiving Day. Your heart will be nourished and your sense of the real meaning of thanksgiving and community will deepen your own celebration.

10. Participate in something fun and physical; many communities have holiday fun walk/runs. Or you could just enjoy a good long walk with the whole family before (or after) dinner. You may find that a good workout before the feast makes you feel less like gorging and more conscious of healthy eating.

Holiday Parties

Rule number 1 is to join in; you'll come to resent your lifestyle if there's no life in it. In the stretch from Thanksgiving through New Year's Eve, parties abound; you will, quite naturally, want to participate in the fun, as well you should. The holiday season is a bright, joyous, hope-filled time of the year, and it does us all good to bask in the warmth of family and good friends. Do so mindful that the real joy of the season is found in fellowship, not on the buffet table. However, it's the latter that will give you a metabolic hangover, so here are some tips to guide your holiday eating pleasures.

1. Don't arrive hungry. Eat something carb-appropriate (and rich in protein) before you go. You usually don't know what's being served, but chances are there will be carbs involved, and arriving hungry at a cocktail buffet or dinner party sets you up to overeat. Some leftover meat or chicken, a hardboiled egg or two, or even just a protein shake can take the edge off your hunger.

2. Limit your intake of beer, wine, and spirits. Enjoy a glass or two, but then move on to seltzer or water. This advice isn't so much about the calories and/or the carbs involved or the dampening effect that too much alcohol has on fat burning—although, to be

sure, those factors figure in—but rather that under the influence of a warm alcohol glow, it's easier to make carb-costly food choices. The more you imbibe, the more likely you'll find yourself saying, "What the hey, sure, I'll have another piece of pie or three."

3. At a cocktail buffet, fill up on the salad, raw veggies, nuts, meats, and cheeses. Steer clear of the breads and crackers if you can. Position yourself in conversation away from the buffet table or at the very least away from the dessert display. Plan to enjoy a bite or two of dessert if you see something you really crave. If you choose to have more, do so knowing what the metabolic effect of overindulgence will be: a blood sugar spike, a rise in insulin levels, and fluid retention by the next morning.

4. Follow each holiday party with a day in Low-Carb Boot Camp, particularly if you went a bit overboard. Several days if you went way overboard.

Develop a Maintenance Mind-set

You've spent many weeks or perhaps even months getting to this point, and the rewards have been worth it: a leaner body; lower readings in blood pressure, blood sugar, cholesterol, or triglycerides; reduction in the risk of cardiovascular diseases; improved sleep patterns; and fewer medications on the shelf. What you've done so far is a wonderful achievement, and you should be proud of your hard work. But everything you've accomplished will have been for nothing if you don't make an ongoing commitment to your new healthy lifestyle.

Maintaining your correction is the name of the game, but never forget that maintenance is a journey, not a destination. The road won't always be easy. Like all of us, you're human; you'll have ups and downs, slips and missteps, but we assure you that none will ever be unrecoverable.

If you sometimes stray from the path, it's pretty simple to find your way back. In this chapter, we've given you the week of meal plans that we call Low-Carb Boot Camp, which will quickly put your metabolic machinery back aright. That will be a surefire recovery system in maintenance, but don't forget that you've already got a good road map. Your original low-carb corrective diet—the one you used to lose weight or correct your health in the first place—will always guide you back to control, no matter how far you stray.

In the months and years ahead, if you find your grasp on health and fitness goals begin to slip, the treatment is simple: make a pact with yourself that you'll go to Boot Camp or return to the corrective level of your plan for a week or two, or however long is necessary, to reestablish control. Go back to the basics, plan and eat the prescribed meals, and carefully record your intake, exercise, and progress. Do it one day at a time, one meal at a time—if necessary, one bite at a time. Accept no excuses from yourself; never say you can't. You can—you already did. And remind yourself that no one has control of what you eat but you. No one.

We wish you the very best health and fitness from now on.

CHAPTER 5

Answers to All Your Low-Carb Questions

In this chapter, we have compiled the most frequently asked questions that relate to low-carb dieting in general, with specific references based on our own Protein Power low-carb philosophy. The questions, gathered from nearly two decades of clinical experience with patients and countless letters from readers, cover all phases of low-carb dieting, not just maintenance. We encourage you to skim through them all, because at some point along the way in your maintenance journey you may experience one or more of these situations. You'll want to turn to this resource again and again for answers to questions that may arise. If you have a question that isn't covered here, please visit our Web site at www. proteinpower.com, where you can post your question. If it is one with broad appeal, we'll post an answer and add it to our question archives. You may also post a question to the Protein Power Bulletin Board, where avid low-carb dieters meet to discuss topics and support one another.

General Questions about the Plan

I have high blood pressure, type 2 diabetes, and increased cholesterol levels, and I am overweight. I take medications for all of my health conditions. How will the diet affect my health problems, and will I be able to stop some of my medications?

You should be quite pleased with the effect. In our experience, as long as people continue to follow the diet, almost two-thirds of people with high blood pressure are able to stop taking medication or at least lower the doses of their blood pressure medicine. Almost 100 percent are able to stop taking their cholesterol-lowering medicines. With the help of their doctors, most people with type 2 diabetes are able to reduce or, in many cases, stop using their oral diabetic medicines. We do not suggest or recommend that you discontinue any of your medications on your own. The effects of the diet can be dramatic.

> *Caution:* If you currently take medication for any of these problems, you will need to work with your physician to monitor your progress. This diet is a powerful tool to correct blood pressure, lower blood sugar, and reduce cholesterol and triglycerides. Do not begin the diet and continue to take your current doses of medication for blood pressure or diabetes. The combined effect will be too strong. Work with your physician, who in short order will be able to reduce or even discontinue medications you currently take for these problems. For your safety, do not attempt to alter doses without the assistance of your doctor.

We have posted a Physician's Information Packet on our Web site at www.proteinpower.com that you may download, print, and take to your physician to help him or her guide your progress.

What is the Protein Power diet?

The plan is a nutritional strategy involving lower levels of carbohydrates, adequate protein, and healthy fat choices that has been used successfully since 1996 by millions of dieters. The plan is divided into three main phases: corrective, transition, and maintenance levels. It is designed to lower and control insulin levels by decreasing the intake of carbohydrates. When carbohydrates are broken down into simple sugars and then absorbed into the bloodstream, insulin, a hormone, is released according to the amount of sugar present. Chronically elevated insulin levels are a major risk factor for many of the diseases of modern civilization, such as obesity, hypertension, high cholesterol, heart disease, gout, reflux, iron overload, and sleep apnea, to mention a few. Seventy-five percent of people release too much insulin in response to carbohydrate intake, and as a result, often fall victim to one or more of these common health problems. The plan is designed to control insulin levels and improve health conditions with nutritious food, offering a balanced diet of lean protein, good-quality fats, and plenty of fruits and vegetables. Limitations occur mainly in the amounts of concentrated starches and sugary foods you'll consume.

What can I expect by following a sensible low-carb diet?

By following the diet as we've designed it, you should experience loss of excess weight and an increase in energy, as well as improvement in insulin-resistant health conditions such as hypertension, high cholesterol and triglyceride levels, gout, gastroesophageal reflux disease, diabetes and hypoglycemia, and sleep apnea. It will also decrease food cravings.

Explain the differences between the corrective (or intervention), transition, and maintenance levels on a low-carb diet.

Those terms, specific to our Protein Power LifePlan diet, are echoed in many other low-carb plans. Whatever they're called, they refer on the one end to the earliest stage of the diet, when there's usually the most restriction, and on the other to the more liberal lifestyle regimen, which was designed not for correcting but for holding your ground, with an intermediate step in-between.

On our Protein Power weight-loss program, for instance, the corrective or intervention phase is the first level to start on the plan; we recommend that everyone new to the low-carb diet start here for at least the first thirty days. Even in people who do not need to lose much weight, this phase will help the body convert into a more efficient fat burner and will allow for the correction of any other insulin-related health problems. The corrective phase consists of eating the proper amount of protein, eating only a small serving of carbohydrates at each meal (which will actually be about 30 grams of effective carbohydrates per day), choosing from healthy fat choices, and drinking at least 2 quarts of water or other noncaloric fluid each day. It also requires that you take additional supplements of magnesium and potassium to replace electrolytes that may be lost during this phase. You should stay at this level until you've almost reached your goals. This corrective level is also the one you can briefly return to during maintenance if you've been on a diet holiday and need to lose a few pounds again.

The next phase, transition, consists of maintaining adequate protein intake for your body's needs as you did during the corrective phase, increasing carbohydrate intake to the moderate level (which works out to about 45 to 50 effective grams a day), and continuing with healthy fat choices. This phase is recommended for people who have reached their health goals and are ready to enjoy eating a few more carbohydrates. Maintenance level is the phase in which you'll increase your carbohydrates to an amount that affords you maximum variety but allows you to still maintain your newly found goal weight and health status. The level of carbohydrates varies for each individual and is partially dependent on how much exercise you do. As with the other levels, adequate protein intake is a must, along with healthy fat choices.

How much magnesium and potassium do I need to take?

Magnesium and potassium are important electrolytes that need to be replaced while you follow the corrective phase of a low-carb diet. Almost 75 percent of people don't even get the RDA of magnesium, a mineral that's critical to more than 300 enzyme systems in the body, and consequently, they begin their diet on the low side. Because a low-carb diet effectively encourages the body to waste excess body fluid, especially in the first few weeks of dieting, these two minerals get lost to a greater degree in the urine and must be replaced.

To start, we recommend that you take 2 over-the-counter magnesium and potassium supplement tablets twice a day with meals. Most OTC tablets contain 99 mg of magnesium and 99 mg of potassium. While some people do fine on this dosage, others may experience looser stools. If this is a problem, reduce the dose to 3 or even 2 tablets per day total.

If you have difficulty finding suitable supplements in your area, you can visit www.proteinpower.com for more information.

A word of caution for patients who take prescription medications for blood pressure or fluid retention: some medications for high blood pressure and fluid can cause you to retain potassium. If you take medications for these conditions, speak to your pharmacist before taking more than 2 OTC potassium pills per day, or, better yet, supplement only if a blood test by your physician shows borderline or low levels of these minerals. Once you've corrected any health problems or neared your ideal weight, you'll move to transition, where you'll slowly increase your carbohydrate intake, first to a moderate serving at each meal or snack and then, in maintenance, to a large serving at each meal or snack. If you choose your carb foods wisely—primarily from a wide variety of fruits and vegetables and not by loading up on empty carbs from refined grains and sugar— you should handle the added carb intake without a problem. You'll also find that the more active you are physically, the larger the amount of carbohydrates you'll be able to handle and not regain weight or see your blood pressure, blood sugar, blood cholesterol, or triglycerides rise again. If you cannot tolerate this increase of carbohydrates, then lower them back down to a moderate level and get your extra calories from healthy meats, fish, poultry, dairy, nuts, and good fats such as those in olives, olive oil, butter, coconut oil, and avocados.

How much weight can I expect to lose on a low-carb plan?

Because everyone is different metabolically, the results will vary. People with a lot to lose will shed more per week than those with very little to lose. Of course, the more compliant you are, the better results you will see. And clearly, adding exercise to your daily routine will help you burn even more calories and improve your cardiovascular picture even further. Women, on average, can expect to lose 2 to 3 pounds per week and men, on average, 3 to 5 pounds per week. That's not to say that in a given week you'll always see 2 to 3 pounds of weight loss. Some weeks may be more, others less. But over the course of the diet, if you take the number of pounds you've lost and divide it by the number of weeks you spent losing it, you should hit close to those averages. Initially, the weight loss will be slightly greater due to the release of excess fluid from tissues. This is one of the first signs that your plan is working to reduce insulin levels. In the first few days, you'll find yourself in the restroom much more often until this loss of excess fluid is complete. Soon, your fluid balance will be stable again and the loss will be primarily from excess fat.

And here's a word to the wise about weighing. It is best not to use the scale as the main indicator of your progress. The scale weighs everything: fat, muscle, and fluid. It can't differentiate between what's in your stomach and what's around your waist. Because fat weighs less than lean mass, you may lose a pound of fat and gain a pound of muscle, but the scale won't show any loss. Focus more on the architecture of your body, its volume, its size, and its shape. To better measure your real progress in fat loss, select an article of clothing—a pair of pants, a fitted skirt, or a belt—and use it each week when you weigh. Then, if the scale fails to show your progress but the belt is another notch in, you can rest assured that you're still losing fat, and this will help to keep your motivation high.

How long after starting the diet should I see results?

Within a few days, the body begins to rid itself of excess retained body fluid; this is one of the first visible signs that the diet is working. Usually within a week energy levels climb, endurance increases, hunger and sugar cravings diminish, and blood pressure begins to normalize. Fat loss begins right away but after week 2, will usually settle into an average 2 to 3 pounds per week for women and 3 to 5 pounds per week for men. Cholesterol and triglyceride levels usually correct within three to six weeks.

How does the Protein Power diet compare to other low-carb diet plans?

Versus Atkins: The Protein Power diet is less restrictive and less extreme than Dr. Atkins's original (and "new") diet revolution, owing to our recognition of the neutral role of fiber and our development of the Effective Carbohydrate Content (a concept adopted by Dr. Atkins in later years as the "net Atkins carb count"). This concept allows for a diet richer and more varied in fruits and vegetables even in the beginning stages of the diet. The Protein Power diet is more mindful of fat quality and even of quantity and of the fact that calories do count, especially for smaller people or those with only small amounts of weight to lose. Protein Power does not focus on ketosis or the technique of dietary fat loading to achieve ketosis in people who are unable to turn their keto strips purple.

Versus the South Beach Diet: Dr. Arthur Agatston, an imaging cardiologist, has, admittedly, come into the diet arena only recently, but he's on the right track—that is, the lowering of carbs for the betterment of health. He's shopped around in various dietary camps and come away with something that's an amalgam of Eades, Atkins, Sears, Sugar Busters, Brand-Miller, and Willet. His diet recommendations are pretty much a variation of Protein Power—reduction of carbohydrates in the first two weeks (which he even calls Phase I, as we did in our book *Protein Power*), then he begins to add small amounts of foods containing sugars and starches (fruits, alcohol, breads, sweets, etc.) in Phase II, and he increases the carbohydrate portions in Phase III. There's not much to set this diet apart from Protein Power except that he still believes in the saturated-fat-is-bad myth (but, oddly, allows red meat and bacon) and aims to keep these "bad" fats from the diet; he also forbids the intake of alcohol, particularly beer, in the early phases of his plan. His reasoning on this point is faulty; he wrongly indicts beer as being filled with the sugar maltose, which it isn't, since virtually all of the digestible carbs in beer are fermented into alcohol. In addition, he endorses the consumption of whole-grain products, such as oatmeal and whole grain bread. In this way, his diet plan is more like the Zone or Dr. Walter Willet's diet.

Versus the Zone: Dr. Sears's Zone is basically a low fat/low calorie diet. It's slightly higher in protein and slightly lower in carbs than the traditional American diet of today, but it's really not a low-carb diet. Followed to the letter, a grown woman of medium build would get about 850 calories a day for life. In addition, the Zone is a complicated regimen, with all the matching up of 30 percent this and 40 percent that with 30 percent of some other thing at each meal or snack. For the average busy person, it's time consuming and tedious and serves no important metabolic purpose. Controlled clinical research in head-to-head trials has shown that a dietary structure almost identical to Protein Power's, while higher in fat and lower in carbs, is more effective at controlling insulin and blood sugar; at reducing triglycerides, total cholesterol, and LDL cholesterol; and at raising HDL cholesterol than is one like the Zone's.

Versus Sugar Busters: This diet, while sort of a low-carb approach, relies heavily on the glycemic index (GI), which is a concept that we don't think has much real-world value and thus don't concern ourselves with it. Again, generally speaking, we have no quarrel with the idea of selecting foods of lower glycemic index. It's a fine idea, but our experience tells us that absolute numbers of effective carb grams are more important when you're trying to lose weight and restore health. Too many carbs, even if they're low GI carbs, won't restore metabolic balance to the seriously resistant individual. For less resistant, more athletic, younger, healthier people, simply eating at the low end of the GI scale may be enough.

Versus Eat Right for Your Blood Type: Only Dr. D'Adamo's type O diet and, to a lesser extent, his type B diet, have much in common with a low-carb diet. Type A is vegetarian and type AB a sort of hybrid. The type O diet cautions against consumption of wheat, gluten, corn, and many other grain and bean lectins and aims to develop a mild metabolic acido-sis in the dieter, factors in common with many lower-carb diets. The structure of the Protein Power diet, on the other hand, encourages the consumption of alkaline fruits and veggies to counterbalance the acidity of meat and cheese, since an ongoing mild metabolic acidosis would pro-mote bone loss. Despite the very authoritative tone of the book, an extensive literature search fails to find much corroboration for his theory. There simply doesn't seem to be any serious scientific correlation between the development of blood types and the response to diet. Infec-tions, yes, but not to diet.

Versus Carbohydrate Addicts: The Hellers' diet is an extremely low-carb diet during most of the day, then it encourages high-carb/high-fat/high-food intake for an hour a day in the Reward Meal. In the long run, we do not feel that it is a means to recover from an addiction, cure insulin-resistance problems, or achieve long-term weight control. We advocate a less stringent approach, but one that is constant all day long, all week long, until the body heals its metabolism and recovers its insulin sensitivity, reduces inflammation, normalizes lipids and blood sugar, and so on. Then we let people indulge in short vacations from their mainte-nance diet for their mental/psychological well-being. To our way of thinking, the reward should be a leaner, healthier body, not a bowl of Rocky Road.

What blood pressure medicines do you use when you need to use one?

ACE inhibitors are our first choice if medication is needed. Calcium channel blockers are also acceptable medications we will sometimes use when we feel that additional medication is necessary along with dietary control. We don't recommend the use of most diuretics (particularly those in the thiazide class) or beta-blockers because they can raise insulin levels.

In your program, do you look at the glycemic index of foods? In other words, do you take into account how much individual foods will raise blood-sugar levels?

Yes and no. In our opinion, the glycemic index isn't a particularly useful tool in the real world. The index is based on how much 100 grams of a given food, eaten alone on an empty stomach, raises blood sugar, as compared to 100 grams of white bread. Based on this index, foods receive a glycemic index number; the higher the number, the more the food raises blood sugar. While it's generally helpful to know this information, people don't normally eat a single food on an empty stomach, then wait to eat the next single food. They eat mixed meals, and the mixing alters the glycemic index. To mainly select foods of a low glycemic index (which most of the foods that we recommend on the Protein Power diet are) is not a bad idea, but there are pitfalls. Fructose, for instance, has a very low glycemic index. Because it has little effect on raising blood sugar or insulin, it has long been recommended as a "good sugar" for people with diabetes. However, the truth is that it actually *promotes* insulin resistance and ultimately worsens blood sugar control.

A refinement to the glycemic index, and a better notion, is the concept of glycemic load, which takes into account both the glycemic index of a food and the size of the serving. This concept is a step forward but still requires that you eliminate from the equation substances like fructose.

Instead of a glycemic index or a glycemic load, we advocate the use of the Effective Carbohydrate Content of foods. This method of counting carbs (total carb content of a food minus the fiber and some portion of the sugar alcohol content) helps people choose healthier foods without worrying about the idea of a good or a bad carbohydrate. It directs people away from potatoes, wheat, refined breads, and pastries and toward the greater nutrition found in a wide variety of greens, colorful vegetables, melons, berries, and other fruit.

I've heard that low-carbohydrate diets cause rapid weight loss of water only. Is that true?

All carb-restricted plans cause a loss of excess retained body fluid in the first week or two through an increased production of urine. This early diuretic effect is one reason why the programs reduce blood pressure so quickly. Most people who struggle with their weight, cholesterol, triglycerides, blood sugar, or blood pressure have high levels of insulin; the excess insulin makes the kidneys retain fluid. The plan lowers insulin levels quickly and simply gets rid of that excess fluid. So, at the beginning of the program you *will* lose some water weight. But after that initial water weight is gone, you'll primarily lose just excess fat week after week. Many of our patients and readers have lost 80, 90, 100 or more pounds. Trust us—it wasn't just water.

Questions about Protein

How do I calculate my protein requirements?

To know how much protein to eat at each meal doesn't require much effort. In *Staying Power* (as well as in our previous book, *The 30-Day Low-Carb Diet Solution*), you'll find tables to guide you to your correct protein serving size—small, medium, large, extra-large, and extra-extra-large. All you have to know is your height and weight and whether you are male or female. What could be simpler?

If you're of a more scientific bent, you may wish to actually calculate your daily protein requirement. It's based on your lean body mass and your activity level. If you want to be really accurate in assessing your lean body mass, you could have a body composition analysis done by a nutritional or fitness professional. That will give you the most accurate lean body mass.

Where can I get an accurate assessment of lean body mass done?

Colleges and universities often offer to their students and even to the public underwater weighing, a hydrostatic body fat test, which is considered the gold standard method. Health clubs, fitness studios, spas, and health providers may offer a bio-impedance or the Tanita method of lean body mass calculation, which relies on the placement of sensor pads or plates on the body or on the soles of the feet to perform a computerized calculation. Other facilities may be expert at the use of fat calipers and can get reliable results that way. If you have access to one of these professional measurement tools, use it by all means. (A word of caution, however; a calculation by calipers or even bio-impedance technology is only as good as the technician doing the measurement. An inexperienced technician may give you a spurious reading.) Remember, too, that it is important to use the same method each time you have a test performed, in order to track your progress.

If you don't have such assessment services available to you, check our book *Protein Power*, where you'll find simple-to-use body composition guidelines that require just a few easy measurements, or visit our Web site at www.proteinpower.com for an interactive calculator based on this model. This method will get you within 1 or 2 percent of the more accurate but less readily available methods of calculating lean mass.

Based on your activity level and your lean body mass in pounds, here's the actual amount of protein you'll require in grams:

Sedentary. A person who gets no physical activity needs 0.5 grams of protein per pound of lean body mass.

Moderately Active. Someone who exercises 20 to 30 minutes two or three times per week needs 0.6 grams of protein per pound of lean body mass.

Active. Someone who exercises 30 minutes or more three to five times per week needs 0.7 grams of protein per pound of lean body mass.

Very Active. A person who exercises an hour or more at least five times per week needs 0.8 grams of protein per pound of lean body mass.

Athlete. A competitive athlete who trains twice a day for an hour or more needs 1 gram of protein per pound of lean body mass.

We also recommend that if people are more than 40 percent overweight, they should increase their protein requirement one level.

What are the best choices of protein-rich foods?

Protein-rich foods come from both animal and plant sources, although animal proteins are far superior in quality. Good sources of protein include all meats, such as beef, lamb, pork, veal, and venison; all poultry, such as chicken, turkey, duck, and so on; and all fish, including shellfish and freshwater and saltwater fish. The category also includes eggs, cheeses (both soft and hard), cottage cheese, and tofu, as well as other soy and nut-based products. And, of course, protein powders from egg or whey are also good sources. Other foods do contain some protein, but we categorize the previous foods as the main protein choices.

How many grams of protein are in each protein choice?

Meats, fish, and poultry = 7 grams of protein per ounce

Eggs = 6 grams for a whole egg, 4 grams per egg white

Hard cheese (formed) = 6–7 grams per ounce

Soft cheese (cream, spreadable)= 3–4 grams per ounce

Curd cheese (cottage, ricotta) = 7 grams per ¼ cup

Tofu = 5 grams per ounce (the firmer it is, the higher in protein content)

What's the difference between hard cheese, soft cheese, and curd cheese?

Hard cheese usually comes in blocks—for example, cheddar, Gouda, Muenster, Swiss, Parmesan, Edam, blue cheese, and mozzarella. Soft cheeses include cream cheese and Neufchatel. Curd cheeses are cottage cheese and ricotta. They differ slightly in the amounts of protein, fat, and carbohydrates they contain.

Is it all right to eat more protein than my recommended amount?

Yes, you can eat more protein if you're still hungry, providing that you don't have existing kidney disease. Your protein intake needs to be monitored more closely in that situation. The amount depends on the size of your lean body mass, but in general, your Protein Requirement is the right portion size. Remember that early man did not have a predictable food supply—one day he might have a feast and then have nothing for days. Our body is flexibly designed to make use of what it can on an irregular schedule, but spreading intake more evenly throughout the day certainly helps to stabilize insulin and blood sugar levels. Remember, too, that eating more protein means eating more calories. If weight loss is a goal for you and you choose to eat a bigger protein serving, you may plateau. In that event, return to the portion we've specified, based on your height and weight.

What happens if I eat less protein than my minimal calculated requirement?

You may not get optimal results from the plan. Your body needs protein to replace wear and tear on its lean tissues, to manufacture enzymes and other important body chemicals, and to support your metabolic rate. If you don't feed your body with enough protein to support your lean mass, your body will perceive the lack as starvation and will behave accordingly: you won't have as much energy and it may be difficult to lose weight. Think of the analogy of a hot, burning fire. The purpose of the fire is to give you heat, and in order to produce heat, you have to fuel the fire with wood. The minute you stop putting wood on the fire, the heat dies out. The body is similar, in that if you put adequate protein and fat into your "furnace," you'll have a higher metabolic rate and therefore more energy. If you put in less protein than your lean mass requires, your furnace won't be able to burn as hot, and, therefore, will produce less energy. Although the fuel your body actually burns is fat or carbohydrates, protein drives the engine.

Does the body store excess protein as fat?

No, not easily or efficiently. Fat is a storage form of energy; the body rarely likes to use protein for energy. It mainly uses protein as raw building material for the production of millions of protein compounds that are needed to replace the wear and tear of daily living. It will, however, easily store excess fat and carbohydrates as fat, but only in the presence of an elevated level of insulin in the blood. As you'll learn in maintenance, it's tough to gain weight even when you're eating lots of protein and fat if you keep your carbs controlled.

Can the body break down muscle mass and turn that protein into carbohydrates?

Yes, if it has to. By reassembling certain amino acids, the liver can manufacture about 200 grams of glucose per day to meet the needs of the few tissues in the body that can burn only glucose for fuel—the red blood cells and certain cells in the eye, kidneys, and brain.

In a state of starvation, the body will break down its own muscle mass to meet this need, but with an adequate amount of dietary protein, it will spare its muscle mass and make glucose from the dietary protein. As long as you keep your dietary protein at or above the recommended minimums on your low-carb plan, your liver will take those proteins and reassemble them into blood sugar as needed in a slow, controlled fashion.

Eating only meat for my protein source gets pretty boring. What can I do about this?

Eating the same thing over and over will become boring no matter what it is. A daily diet of nothing but hot fudge sundaes would grate on the palate over time. That's why we have always encouraged eating a wide variety of foods, both those that mainly contribute to your protein intake and the fruits and vegetables that provide color, texture, and interest. Protein doesn't have to be just meat. Beyond that, it doesn't have to be just eggs, fish, tofu, and cheese. Take a look at the transition and maintenance meal plans in this book (as well as those in *The 30-Day Low-Carb Diet Solution* and the mix-and-match meals in our *Protein Power Life-Plan*). You'll see that we've provided you with varied meals to add some spice to your dining. You can continue to mix and match those meals throughout your life, adding more carb servings as your health and fitness improve.

If you like to cook, you may want to get a copy of our *Low-Carb Comfort Food Cookbook*, which will allow you to bring back whole classes of foods you thought you'd left behind when you went low-carb. You can enjoy high-protein, lower-carb versions of pasta, pizza, or Mexican enchiladas at dinner. Boredom won't be a problem any longer.

There's a wealth of culinary resources available now for the low-carb dieter. You'll find more than 80 recipes in our original *Protein Power* book and nearly one hundred recipes in *The 30-Day Low-Carb Diet Solution,* all of which you can use again and again in your maintenance journey. Along with those options, the steady increase of good low-carb cookbooks in the stores, the explosion of new online resources, and the recipes you can learn on our new PBS cooking show *Low-Carb Cook-woRx* should put variety back onto your plate. Learning to be creative is one of the opportunities of this plan.

What can I eat for breakfast besides eggs?

For a quick meal on the run, a protein shake is a good breakfast alternative and can be made with strawberries, frozen mixed berries, a peach, a kiwi, an orange, or any low-sugar fruit you enjoy. You could also have a protein drink made with a pure protein powder. We recommend a powder that has at least 20 grams of protein and no more than 2 to 3 grams of carbohydrates per serving. Whey protein is the best choice of powders; it has a clean, pleasant taste, and it's very good for your immune system. Egg protein is also biologically complete and easy to absorb. If you cannot use whey or egg, you can use soy or rice protein powder or even spirulina powders, although we'd caution that a growing body of evidence questions the healthfulness of processed soy proteins, which would include soy powders. If you mix the powder with milk, be sure to count the carbohydrates that the milk contributes, as well as the carbohydrates in any fruit that you use.

In our *Low-Carb Comfort Food Cookbook*, you'll find delicious recipes for high-protein, low-carb versions of waffles, pancakes, muffins, Danish, and quick breads. Make a batch of waffles to freeze, then pop them in the toaster for a quick breakfast, topped with low-carb syrup and butter. Make a dozen muffins to freeze, and reheat them for a breakfast on the run.

Sliced hardboiled eggs with cheese melted over low-carb toast (6 grams of effective carbohydrates or less) or Melba toast is another alternative. Yes, we realize that this is an egg dish, but at least it's one that you can prepare mostly in advance and quickly throw together in the morning with little or no cleanup.

A cup of plain yogurt with protein powder mixed in and raw nuts sprinkled on top works well.

You can always have a broiled, lean hamburger, salmon burger, or turkey-burger patty along with fruit (being careful to stay within your carb recommendation). Who says we shouldn't have burgers for breakfast! Low-carb versions of protein bars, hot and cold cereals, as well as muffin, pancake, and waffle mixes, are becoming more available on the market. You can locate these products at your grocer, your local health food store, or online at low-carb specialty stores.

Do you have any suggestions for using leftover egg yolks?

If used right away, say within a day or two, the yolks can be used to make homemade hollandaise sauce, mayonnaise, or low-carb crème brulee. Store them in an airtight container in the refrigerator. If you want to avoid the worry of what to do, you can purchase pasteurized egg whites in the dairy case of your supermarket.

Are there people who should avoid red meat and eggs?

Yes, although not commonly so. A few people fall into this category; some individuals with hypertension, elevated cholesterol, fluid retention, or inflammatory problems such as arthritis, bursitis, asthma, allergies, and rashes may be sensitive to these foods. Usually, these exceptionally sensitive individuals will still lose weight just fine, but their elevated blood pressure, cholesterol, or asthma won't correct until they stop eating the red meat and eggs. See the following question for more information.

Specific Issues

Can I really eat all the red meat and egg yolks I want?

Most people can. However, there are a few concerns to keep in mind. First, you can't do the low-carb diet halfway. You can't increase your protein foods haphazardly and continue to eat carbohydrates as you like and expect to see results. In fact, you'll worsen your problems if you do so.

Second, a few people may have sensitivities to large amounts of these and other foods. These people are often those who have elevated blood pressure and/or cholesterol, retain abnormally high amounts of fluid, and/or suffer from inflammatory conditions such as skin rashes, asthma, allergies, bursitis, or arthritis. The mechanisms causing such sensitivities are quite complex.

In addition, the methods of cooking these foods can be part of the problem. Charring meats to well done and beyond and scrambling egg yolks until they're hard can damage the cholesterol and the fats, turning them into truly harmful substances that may worsen certain health problems.

Here is the strategy for these folks to follow: first, alter the cooking methods. Don't char meat; cook it on the grill to no more than medium. Hard boil, soft boil, or poach eggs or even fry them in butter or olive oil instead of scrambling them.

If these measures don't help, eliminate red meat and egg yolks from your diet completely for three weeks. At the end of the three-week period, take stock of your health. Has it improved? Eat a large portion of red meat and eggs for a couple of meals, and observe what happens. If your problems reappear or get worse, you may indeed be sensitive to arachidonic acid or to the damaged cholesterol and fats from overcooking them. Treat yourself to these foods only once in a while. When you do have them, make sure to remove as much of the fat from the beef as possible. Grill—but don't char—the beef. This will reduce the arachidonic acid by as much as 35 percent. Another option is to marinate the meat in a combination of red wine and olive oil or light sesame oil for twenty-four hours before grilling. This may help to remove some of the arachidonic acid.

As far as eggs are concerned, if you're sensitive to them, have no more than one or two whole eggs at a sitting, don't routinely scramble them, and eat egg whites the rest of the time.

Questions about Carbohydrates

Which foods are classified as carbohydrates?

Carbohydrates come primarily from plant foods: the cereal grains, such as wheat, oats, rice, corn, rye, spelt, and so on; all soy products; all nuts; as well as all vegetables and fruits. There are some carbohydrates in dairy products, and, of course, sugar, honey, molasses, maple syrup, and corn syrup are sources of pure, quickly absorbable, nearly 100 percent carbohydrates. Some carbohydrate foods contain more sugar than others. Be careful with starchy fruits, such as bananas and most other tropical fruits, root veggies, such as potatoes and yams; dried beans and field peas; and all cereal grains. All of these foods break down into simple sugars, which get absorbed into the intestinal tract and then trigger an insulin response. Making appropriate carbohydrate choices is key to your success on a low-carb diet. For example, a medium-sized potato contains starch that your body will break down into about ¼ cup of sugar. A medium-sized tomato, which has much more fiber and other nutrients than it does sugar, will break down into only about 1 teaspoon of sugar. For more information on this topic, refer to the FAQs about the Effective Carbohydrate Content of foods.

How many carbohydrates am I allowed on a sensible low-carb diet, such as the Protein Power diet?

We suggest that everyone striving to lose weight or control weight-related health issues initially start at a small carbohydrate serving with each meal or snack. That's about 7 to 10 effective carbohydrate grams per meal or a total of 30 grams of effective carbohydrates per day. This is the corrective phase carbohydrate intake. Carbohydrates can be spread throughout the day; we recommend that initially you never eat more than a small serving (about 7–10 grams) at one sitting. More than this amount will trigger a higher insulin response, which will then lower blood glucose levels and cause you to crave even more carbohydrates. If you don't use your carbohydrate quota for one meal, you cannot roll it over to the next meal. This again will cause too high of an insulin response. The idea behind controlling the amount of carbohydrates you take in throughout the day is to control your blood glucose and insulin levels throughout the day and allow you to achieve metabolic healing. As your diet changes from transition to maintenance, your carbohydrate intake will increase.

What do you mean when you say effective carbohydrate content?

It means the carbohydrates in any food that can be absorbed by the digestive tract and that cause an elevation of blood sugar and insulin. Generally speaking, effective carbohydrate content (ECC) refers to the sugars and starches in a food.

How is the ECC determined?

On a nutrition label, which is on every packaged food product, you'll find the total carbohydrate content of the food, usually the sugar content, the fiber content, and sometimes the sugar alcohol content and a category called "other starches." The total carbohydrate content is the sum of all the carb sources listed. You can easily determine the effective carbohydrate content of a food by taking the total carbohydrate content and subtracting from it the fiber portion (and about one-third to one-half of the sugar alcohol portion, if present). Neither soluble nor insoluble fiber is absorbed as carbohydrate by the human GI tract and should not be counted as a carbohydrate for the purpose of weight loss, blood-sugar elevations, and insulin response. To be perfectly correct, soluble fiber, while not broken down and absorbed as glucose in the human small intestine, can be acted on by the bacteria in the colon to produce butyric acid and other short-chain fatty acids, which serve to nourish the colon's lining cells. So soluble fiber may contribute calories but not effective carb grams.

The carbohydrates that need to be counted toward your daily intake are the "effective" carbohydrates, or ECC—the amount that will trigger a sugar and insulin response. For most purposes, that means the sugars and starches only, although we would suggest at least counting some portion (say 3 grams of every 10 grams on the label) of any sugar alcohol, at least during the corrective phase, to minimize their over-consumption.

How important is it to follow the correct amount of carbohydrate intake per meal/day as I begin a low-carb plan? What if I eat more carbohydrates?

There's no doubt that the closer you follow the program, the better results you'll get. We've tried cutting carbohydrates back incrementally and slowly bringing them down, and what we've found is that this doesn't do the job very well. When you want to correct an insulin problem, the very best thing you can do is to cut the carbs sharply back, get the insulin controlled, let the metabolic hormones stabilize, and then go from there. As you get everything corrected, you can add the carbs back in slowly. Then, once you approach your goal—whether it's a weight goal, a body-fat goal, cholesterol or triglyceride reductions, or some other health goal—move up to the transition level, and if you remain stable for a few weeks, move on to maintenance. That carbohydrate level will be substantially higher than the one that you used to correct your problems in the first phase. If you overindulge at a meal or two, it won't ruin your corrective plan, but if you do so consistently, you will defeat the purpose of the plan and your progress will stall.

Will I lose weight faster if I just cut out all carbohydrates altogether? Would it be dangerous?

Actually, it wouldn't be dangerous at all in the short run. A number of societies thrive without many carbohydrates. Australian Aborigines live in the desert and eat mainly a meat diet because there isn't a lot of plant food available. Traditional Eskimos get almost no plant material in their diet and little or no carbohydrates. They sometimes do suffer bone loss over a lifetime but not in the short run. Studies have shown that bone loss doesn't occur at all on a meat-based diet that also includes fruits and vegetables to balance the protein and fat. Meat, fish, eggs, and cheese cause an acid load on the body that over decades can weaken bones.

Before you get spooked about the wisdom of low-carb dieting, recognize that all breads, pastas, and cereal grains cause the same acid load that meat and hard cheese do; you won't spare your bones by going meat-free and filling up on bagels and oatmeal. The key is striving to balance the acid load with alkaline foods—fruits, green leafy veggies, colorful veggies, or alkaline waters. That's one reason why we designed our Protein Power strategy as we did—to give you a balance of acid and alkaline foods to keep your bones strong and healthy.

On the other hand, with regard to the metabolism, human biochemistry is designed to do very nicely without carbohydrates, by making them from other things. If we don't get protein, we die. If we don't get fat, we die. If we don't get carbohydrates, nothing much happens, at least in the short run. And that's why it doesn't make sense to go on a high-carbohydrate diet at the expense of fat and protein requirements. When we increase our carbohydrate intake and cut back on proteins and fats, we're taking in lots of a substance that nature gave us the biochemistry to manufacture in our bodies, and missing out on things we can't make. So as far as not eating any carbohydrates, yes, you could, but you'd miss out on good sources of balancing alkaline foods, miss out on some of the phytochemicals and antioxidants found in plant foods that you need to be truly healthy, and miss out on the variety that will make it easy to stick to your plan for life.

Do I have to spread out my carbohydrate intake throughout the day or can I just save them all up and eat them all at once?

You really can't save them up, unfortunately. Carbohydrates have an expiration date with each meal—particularly during the corrective phase. There's a metabolic impact to eating carbohydrates. If you eat a small serving, you'll raise your insulin a little bit. If you eat a large serving, you'll raise it more. For instance, if you've saved up all 30 grams allotted during the corrective phase or the 80 to 100 grams or more that you may tolerate during maintenance and you eat them all at one time, you'll experience a greater metabolic impact—your insulin will really go up. When that happens, it's like climbing right back on the insulin roller coaster. Up goes the insulin, down goes the blood sugar, and then up go the hunger and the cravings. You really do yourself more harm than good when you try to save up carbohydrates and use them all at one time.

If you plan to eat a bit more carbohydrates than normal, the time to do it is in the morning. Insulin receptors are more effective in the morning than they are later in the day. They actually move sugar out of the blood more quickly with less insulin.

What are good bread choices while on the corrective level of carbohydrate intake?

It's challenging to incorporate traditional breads at a small serving of fewer than 10 grams of carbohydrates per meal, although the ever-increasing number of low-carb products entering the marketplace certainly makes that easier to do. Although most of these products still have a way to go in the taste and texture departments, they're getting better. Begin to explore the many low-carb food stores popping up around the country, cruise the low-carb offerings in the grocery store, and check out low-carb sites on the Internet, where you'll find many new bread options. For instance, the advent of tasty low-carb tortillas has been a big boon to the scene.

With all pre-packaged products, be sure to read the labels carefully. And remember: *caveat emptor!* Let the buyer beware. Low-carb labeling laws are still in flux, and what you see there may not be a totally correct representation of carb truth. If it tastes too good to be true, it may be, and it would behoove you to investigate the ingredients a little further.

For many people, however, it may be easier to avoid most of the grain-based products while on the corrective phase and slowly add them to your diet when you move to the transition level, where your serving will give you about 15 grams of carbs per meal. Your Small Serving in the Carbohydrate Servings Lists in appendix B in this book and in *The 30-Day Low-Carb Diet Solution,* will guide you to acceptable choices.

Are fruits and vegetables eliminated on this diet or are they restricted?

Even on the most restrictive phase of a sensible low-carb plan, you'll see a big selection of fruits and veggies scaled for the small carb-serving size. Just as was the case in *Protein Power, Protein Power LifePlan,* and *The 30-Day Low-Carb Diet Solution,* your *Staying Power* meal plans include fruits and vegetables at every meal and most snacks. You'll probably eat more servings of fruits and veggies on this plan than on any diet you've ever tried—at least, on any one that worked!

Using the effective carbohydrate content (ECC) concept, you can incorporate a wide variety of fruits and vegetables into your plan. You can eat a chef salad that is so big you can't eat the whole thing and not even come close to exceeding your carbohydrate limit—as long as you make the right choices. The whole idea that effective low-carbohydrate diets don't contain fruits and vegetables (or don't contain very many) is a myth. It may have been true in the past before people understood how to subtract the fiber to get the effective carbohydrate content. Back in the old low-carbohydrate diet days, you basically had meats and cheeses and not much room for fruits and vegetables. On almost all of the second-generation carb-controlled diets, you'll get plenty of fruits and vegetables—probably more than you're able to eat.

Many low-carb bars contain sugar alcohols. What are they and how do I account for them in my carbohydrate totals?

We address this topic in several spots in this chapter, but it's an important one. These sweeteners are classified as neither sugars nor alcohols, but they're carbohydrates nonetheless. Examples include glycerin, maltitol, mannitol, xylitol, lactitol, erythrotol, sorbitol, and others. Whereas they once turned up only in sugar-free chewing gum and some diabetic specialty candies, the low-carb product revolution that's swept the nation has caused an explosion of sugar alcohols in foods ranging from breakfast bars and chocolate bars to pancake syrup and barbecue sauce, to ice cream and brownies.

At the present time, they have not been legally classified for product-labeling purposes, as are sugars, starch, and fiber, although more and more they are treated as "other carbohydrates" on labels. Some manufacturers choose to omit them from the total carb count in the nutrient data panel of the label (they must, however, declare the amount of sugar alcohol in the ingredient list). Because sugar alcohols aren't actually sugar, products that contain them may use the term *sugar free* on the label.

There are some claims that sugar alcohols don't have usable carbs and therefore don't count; that they can be completely subtracted if listed on the label. This statement is not entirely false, but it is misleading. Sugar alcohols do have carbs, but the carbs they contain are more slowly and incompletely absorbed from the small intestine than sugar is, thus producing a much smaller and slower rise in blood sugar and consequently insulin.

What's the effective carb content of sugar alcohols? At this point, their ECC hasn't been determined clearly. A rule of thumb might be to count 2 to 3 grams for every 10 grams on the label, but that's really just a ballpark estimate and depends not just on the sugar alcohol in question but on the person consuming it. We'd recommend that you use them sparingly, watch your progress in weight loss or health correction, and if progress stalls, cut back on or cut out your use of sugar alcohols.

The sugar alcohols don't all behave the same. For instance, glycerin seems to elevate blood sugar in people with type 1 diabetes (those who must take insulin shots) more than the sugar alcohols do. Beware of overeating sugar alcohols. They have a laxative effect, which happens for two reasons: first, the sugar alcohols are not completely absorbed, and they hold onto a lot of water in the bowel. This causes diarrhea. Another consequence is unpleasant gas and bloating. Sorbitol and mannitol are the worst offenders in this department, xylitol and maltitol less so. Xylitol, which is now commercially available to the consumer, seems to be less absorbed and for some people to cause less GI tract discomfort.

In general, some people tolerate many sugar alcohols well, while others can't stomach even a bit of any of them. For those who seem to tolerate their intake, what indeed does that mean? If they don't suffer GI upset and diarrhea from consuming a sugar alcohol, does that imply that they're absorbing it more effectively? And if so, should those absorbed grams be counted, and as what? Carbs? Alcohol? Calories? The issue of sugar alcohols will plague us for a while until it all gets sorted out. In the meantime, our advice: use caution! If a product contains more than 2 or 3 grams of any sugar alcohol, eat just a small amount and assess your own response to it. Keep in mind that the GI effect of sugar alcohols will add up; a couple of grams in syrup, a couple of grams in jam, a couple of grams in ice cream, and a couple of grams in a few pieces of candy add up to a lot of couples and potentially an unpleasant GI effect. And, remember, carb content aside, they do have calories—about one-half to three-quarters the calories of an equal number of grams of sugar. So they're not a "free food."

Questions about Fats

Which foods are classified as fats?

Healthy fat sources are found in nuts, seeds, nut butters, avocados, olives, olive oils, butter, fresh fish oils, flax seeds and fresh flaxseed oil, as well as in the fat in natural meats, poultry, and game. The fats to avoid are partially hydrogenated fats; trans-fats, found in fast foods and in most boxed or prepackaged foods with a shelf life; most types of shortening and margarine; foods that are deep-fried in polyunsaturated vegetable oils; and nuts that have been heated to high temperatures (canned). Many foods contain fats, as well as carbohydrates and protein.

How much fat is allowed on a low-carb diet?

Obviously, that depends on the diet, because there are some differences. With the exception of *Enter the Zone* and to some extent *The South Beach Diet*, most low-carb plans, including ours, do not focus on the amount of fat. We focus on quality more than on quantity. Initially, fats are not counted into your daily caloric intake. Healthful fats do not trigger an insulin response, so they're not a threat to insulin-resistance problems, but they do trigger the release of an enzyme in the stomach, cholecystokinin (CCK), which sends signals to the satiety center in the brain, telling us that we're full. Fats do, however, account for 9 calories per gram, so excess fat intake can hinder weight loss. Be sensible about your fat intake. If you hit a plateau, then you may need to lower your fat intake—or raise your activity output.

I have heard that flaxseed oil is a good source of omega-3 oils. What are your recommendations?

Since writing *Protein Power* in 1996, we have modified our viewpoint on flaxseed oils. While it's true that people who are ill or have diabetes may not be able to effectively convert flaxseed oil into the essential fats that are found ready-made in fish oils, most people can benefit from fresh flaxseeds or fresh flaxseed oil, in addition to fish oils. Both contain high amounts of omega-3 oils. We still believe that good-quality fresh fish oil is preferable, as long as it's pure and toxin free, although with growing concerns about toxins, such as mercury and PCBs, in our fish supply, flaxseed oil may be a good choice for those of us healthy enough to make the conversion.

Omega-3 fatty acids are a family of long-chain polyunsaturated fats whose members share a unique chemical structure. These fats are incorporated into virtually all the cells of the body and, among other tasks, form potent hormonelike structures called eicosanoids. Eicosanoids are believed to play a significant role in boosting the immune response and influencing conditions as varied as arteriosclerosis, cancer, inflammatory conditions, and allergic reactions. The adult daily recommendation for omega-3 fatty acids is estimated to be 300 to 400 mg per day.

Which foods contain saturated fats? Are they harmful?

Saturated fats come primarily from animal sources and certain tropical plants. The term *saturated* refers to their having every carbon in their chemical structure fully surrounded by hydrogen ions. This configuration is quite stable, not easily damaged by oxygen, heat, or chemical reactions. Saturated fats are found in meats, poultry, game, dairy, and eggs, as well as in coconut oil and palm kernel oil. Saturated fats from these sources usually pose no problems in a diet that also includes unsaturated oils from such foods as olives, nuts, avocados, and fish. Foods such as bacon, sausage, hot dogs and other processed meat products, and yellow cheeses are usually higher in saturated fats than are meats from wild game; leaner cuts of beef, such as top sirloin, flank steak, and New York steak; or poultry.

Although eating fattier foods is not a problem for most people who follow a balanced low-carb approach, for a few people, excess saturated fats may slow their progress toward weight and health goals. We recommend that you choose a wide variety of the foods available to you on your plan—don't allow yourself to fall into a rut of eating just burgers, hot dogs, and eggs and bacon every day. Be sure to include some healthier fats from plant sources, such as raw nuts and nut butters, avocados, olives and olive oil, grape seed oil, and omega-3 fish oils, found in coldwater fish such as salmon (preferably wild), mackerel, albacore tuna, sardines, and herring.

Are nuts a healthy choice?

Nuts are a good, portable source of high-quality fats and protein that have been available to us since hunter-gatherer times. Most of them do have a few grams of usable carbohydrate, which you should be sure to account for in your daily totals while you are in the corrective or the transition phase. True nuts—such as almonds, macadamia nuts, pistachios, pecans, walnuts, pinyon nuts, Brazil nuts, and cashews—all offer a healthful source of calories. Peanuts—America's staple nut—are not really nuts at all but rather legumes, in the same category as dried beans and field peas. They are higher in starch and more likely than real nuts to stimulate allergy problems. While it's fine to eat peanuts on occasion, we'd recommend that you choose nuts of better quality most of the time.

Use nuts to snack on or to add to foods. They're an especially good snack when you are in maintenance. Raw nuts or dry roasted nuts are the best choice, since they haven't been cooked in poor-quality oils. If you experience allergic problems from raw nuts, which is not uncommon, try roasting the raw nuts yourself at low temperatures in the oven or lightly toasting them in a skillet. Watch them closely, shake them often, and don't let them burn!

Should I use mayonnaise? Light mayonnaise? Reduced-fat butter?

Finding a good-quality mayonnaise can be a challenge. If you can find one made from good-quality oil, not partially hydrogenated soybean oil or any other partially hydrogenated oil—go for it. Unfortunately, such choices are not widely available. In years past, we recommended that you purchase canola oil mayonnaise, which you can easily find at most health food markets, but recent evidence suggests that the deodorizing process necessary to make canola oil odor-free and tasty also damages the fats in it, converting some of them to unhealthful transfats. We no longer recommend the use of canola oil for cooking, in salad dressings, or in mayonnaise. If you rarely use mayonnaise, it probably doesn't matter much what product you use, as long as it's a real mayonnaise—a little touch of something not so good probably won't hurt. However, if you love to slather on the mayo, your best choice is to make your own real mayonnaise from high-quality oil. It's really quite easy to make mayonnaise in the blender. You'll find our recipe for quick real mayonnaise using light olive oil in the recipe section of *The 30-Day Low-Carb Diet Solution*, as well as in our *Low-Carb Comfort Food Cookbook* and on our TV cooking show Web site at www.lowcarbcookworx.com. You could also use any true nut oil, sesame oil, or avocado oil to make mayonnaise. The type of oil you pick will color the flavor of the mayonnaise.

As far as butter goes, use real sweet cream unsalted butter. The fats in butter are mainly short- and medium-chain triglycerides, which you can use readily for quick energy.

Combination Foods: Nuts, Dairy, Condiments, Dressings, and Alcohol

How do I count foods such as milk, yogurt, and dairy foods? Are they fats, protein, or carbohydrates?

Milk and plain yogurt are what we call combination foods. They contain both protein and carbohydrates and, except in nonfat varieties, some fat as well. A cup of milk or yogurt (we call them fluid dairy products) contains approximately 12 to 13 grams of carbohydrate and 8 to 9 grams of protein. This number of carb grams would exceed the small serving level of carbohydrates and take you beyond your carb limit for a meal during the corrective phase of your plan. A 4-ounce portion, however, would fit in just fine. If you love milk or yogurt, simply cut back on the portion size per meal until you're ready to move toward maintenance.

Should I count cottage cheese as protein or carbohydrates?

Both. You will want to count the protein in cottage cheese as a healthy contribution to your protein intake (7 grams per ¼ cup). It's a great alternative breakfast choice to eggs and bacon now and again. Pair it with some wedges of fresh tomato or with a half cup of low-sugar fruits, such as strawberries or blueberries. But you must remember that all real dairy products also contain some carbohydrates from the lactose in milk. Cottage cheese has 2 grams of carbohydrate per ¼ cup—that works out to about 1 gram per ounce. That's pretty much in the same range as all dairy products: hard and soft cheeses have a bit less than 1 gram per ounce, and fluid dairy products have about 1½ grams of carbohydrate per ounce. The availability of carb-reduced dairy products has changed the landscape somewhat, making a full 8-ounce serving of milk possible in the corrective phase of dieting.

How do you count nuts? As a protein, a carbohydrate, or a fat?

Most nuts have a fair amount of protein and fat, as well as some carbohydrates. Remember, as long as you're losing (or not gaining) weight, you don't count fat, and your protein requirement is a minimum, not a fixed, amount, so unless you have trouble meeting your daily protein requirement for some reason you don't have to worry about the protein or fat content of the nuts. Just count the effective grams of carbohydrate in your daily total. Among the true nuts, macadamia nuts have the best profile because almost all their carbohydrates are fiber—very little carb is left to raise insulin levels. The drawback, of course, is expense. We used to joke with our patients that they could eat all the macadamia nuts they could afford.

What condiments can I use on the plan?

You can use any condiment as long as you count the carbohydrates. Some condiments tend to be fairly high in carbs, such as BBQ sauces, ketchup, and some salad dressings. You may choose not to trade those precious carb grams for such a small amount of food. Just read the labels carefully to help you decide. More and more tasty low-carb condiments are now available commercially. Look for them in health food and natural groceries and online. You can find recipes for low-carb salad dressings, sauces, marinades and rubs, and mayonnaise in many low-carb cookbooks, including ours.

Can I drink alcohol on a low-carb diet?

Although on some plans, such as *The South Beach Diet*, the answer is no, as far as we're concerned, on ours you can! But only within the limit of your carbohydrate maximum. As a rule of thumb, dry white or red wine (3 oz.) or light beers (12 oz.) will cost you 3 or 4 effective carb grams, but they are still reasonable choices as long as you count them in your daily totals. Hard liquor will cost you a lot of empty calories, so take it easy. Wine—in moderation—can even help improve insulin sensitivity and is good for your cardiovascular health, so enjoy. Be sensible with your intake; alcohol is one place where just because a little is good, that doesn't mean a lot is better.

Potential Side Effects of Low-Carb Diets

What follows is a discussion of some potential mild side effects that may occur when you start a low-carb diet. The recommendations are general and are intended as a basic first-line guide and not as a substitute for your doctor. In each and every case, if the symptom persists, you should visit your doctor.

I just started the program, and I'm feeling a little weak and tired. Why is that?

This is not uncommon when you first start on the program. We always tell our patients not to do anything too strenuous for a few days until they adjust to the new diet. It takes a little time to make the enzymes that are needed to adapt to a lower-carbohydrate diet. Enzymes are what our bodies make to cause all the chemical reactions that go on in the body. When we start a new type of diet that requires new enzymes to make it work, it takes a few days for those enzymes to get produced by the body. Until that happens, your body still thinks it's back on a high-carbohydrate diet. When your body adapts, you'll have more endurance and you'll feel a lot better.

People sometimes experience a feeling as if they're out of gas in the first few days. If you feel that slump or if you feel hungry, don't try to solve it by going out and eating carbohydrates. You'll just put yourself behind the eightball again. If you're going to eat, eat extra protein and fat. Eat things like nuts, seeds, or olives. Deli meat, hard-boiled eggs, deviled eggs, or leftover steak, fish, or chicken are also good choices. These are all good alternatives to quickly get protein and fat into your diet and give you a little "pick me up" without disrupting the metabolic harmony you're trying to achieve.

Finally, be sure that you're taking a potassium-magnesium supplement. Forgetting to take potassium in the early days of the plan is the single most common reason for side effects. Take your potassium! You can get a suitable over-the-counter product containing 99 mg of potassium and 99 mg of magnesium per tablet at most health food stores or vitamin shops. Take 3 or 4 of these a day during the corrective phase of low-carb dieting. If you can't find a product near you, check our Web site at www.proteinpower.com.

What should I do if I feel dizzy or lightheaded?

Sometimes that happens—it can happen on any diet. On this particular diet, in the first few days or the first week especially, your loss of fluid (and with it potassium and sodium) can sometimes make you feel a little bit dizzy or lightheaded.

Any time you feel dizzy, increase your fluid intake and be sure to take your potassium and magnesium. If you've been taking it all along, you may want to consider raising the intake level just a little bit. We recommend taking on average 200 to 600 mg of each magnesium and 200 to 400 mg of potassium daily in divided doses. Be aware that excess magnesium will cause diarrhea, so increase your dose slowly. Add a little bit of sodium to your diet. This is probably the only time you're ever going to hear a doctor say to add sodium to your diet, but in this case you might need to. As your insulin level falls rapidly, sometimes you release excess fluid a little too quickly, so you may need to add a small amount of sodium. In the summertime it's especially important. If you're outside working in the yard or you're exercising and sweating a lot, you'll lose sodium and potassium. On a low-carb diet, if you start to feel a little dizzy, one thing you may want to do to increase your sodium is to eat salty foods—dill pickles or olives, for example—or drink a cup of bouillon. Although you may be more familiar with doctors advising you not to eat salt, this is a different situation, and in this instance, eating a little bit of extra sodium not only isn't harmful, it may be helpful. Just don't overdo it.

I've been experiencing chronic headaches since I started on the plan. What should I do?

The first thing you should do is to drink more water every day. Make sure that you're taking at least the recommended amount of potassium and magnesium. You may even need to take an extra tablet. If you have not seen any improvement, you might want to check your ketone levels. You can get a product called Ketostix at most drugstores. Just follow the instructions for use. If your ketone level is high—that is, the stick turns dark purple—you may want to try gradually increasing your carbohydrate intake. Some people produce ketones heavily on a lower-carb plan, and this can cause headaches. If you're in heavy ketosis and having headaches or sleeplessness, you'll definitely want to adjust your carbohydrate level up slightly to alleviate the problem. Be sure to do this gradually. Increase carbohydrates by no more than an extra small serving of carbs at breakfast and, if needed, at lunch until the headaches go away. It's important that you continue to limit your carbs as much as possible— but if you develop a persistent headache, that may mean for the short run eating a slightly higher amount of carbs. Although headaches can occur because of heavy ketosis, remember that headache is a common symptom and its cause may be totally unrelated to the diet. Any significant headache that fails to respond to a slight increase in carbohydrates and fluid intake probably merits a visit to your doctor.

I was feeling fabulous but all of a sudden I feel exhausted and my legs are starting to ache, and I have muscle cramps. Should I be concerned?

This describes an almost textbook case of hypokalemia, or low potassium levels. We can't stress enough the importance of taking potassium. The vast majority of problems that people have with this program occur because they don't take their potassium. If you're taking over-the-counter potassium, take at least 4 tablets (at 99 mg each) per day. This program has a strong diuretic effect on the kidneys, and potassium is unavoidably lost in the fluid the kidneys release. If you feel weird at all— if you experience lightheadedness, tingling, fatigue, deep muscle fatigue, muscle aches, or cramps—you're probably low on potassium. Symptoms of low potassium usually occur about a week or so into the diet. If it does happen, we recommend that you use Morton's light salt or No Salt (which is a potassium substitute or a potassium salt) to salt your food. And make sure you take your potassium and magnesium supplements every day as directed. By all means, if the symptoms continue, you really should see your doctor and get your potassium level checked.

I'm having trouble sleeping. Does that have something to do with the diet?

Most people find that they actually sleep a lot better when they go on this program. Very few have problems of sleeplessness, and when they do, excess production of ketones—a by-product of fat breakdown—is usually the cause. The good news is that this means you're getting rid of body fat; the bad news is that heavy ketosis can occasionally cause sleeplessness or a jittery feeling. If you're producing and releasing a lot of ketones, you may have this problem. You can determine ketone levels in your urine by using Ketostix strips, which can be purchased at any pharmacy. Check your ketones in the evening and if the stick turns deep pink to purple, this could be the cause of your sleeplessness. In this case, you should increase your carbohydrate intake a little bit in the evening and drink more water. If you're in the corrective phase, on small carbohydrate servings, you could move up to a moderate serving at dinner or move your snack to the evening to somewhat reduce the level of ketones in your blood during the night. You might also exercise more to use up the ketones.

I have a funny taste in my mouth and have bad breath. Why?

Although, unlike the Atkins diet approach, our program doesn't aim to put you into heavy ketosis, any time you break down fat on a lower-carb diet some degree of ketosis will occur. All of us produce ketones to some extent overnight as we sleep; their production is perfectly natural. When we restrict carbohydrates, we tend to make a few more ketones, which are nothing but a natural by-product of burning fat. But that's fine. Our body deals with them. The body gets rid of ketones in a number of ways; one way is to burn them up. But when we're producing a few more than we're able to burn up, we get rid of the excess mainly in our urine. Some of it goes out through the stool, and some of it goes out through the breath. When excess ketones come out through the breath, they give the mouth a funny taste or what's perceived as bad or fruity-smelling breath—what all low-carbers know as ketone breath. It's very easy to correct. You can increase your carbohydrates just a little bit or exercise more until it goes away. You can also drink lots and lots of water or other noncaloric fluid so that you carry more ketones away in the urine. Or you can use some sort of breath freshener. But you have to be careful about using too many mints, because some of them have a fair amount of sugar. Read the label! Ketone breath is usually a problem only in the early phases of the program. After you get going and you adapt, it tends to go away.

Will I be constipated on this program? If so, what can I do about it?

If you spend your carbohydrate grams on foods that are really high in fiber and high in phytochemicals, you shouldn't be constipated. If you're not a big fiber eater, you might relieve the problem with over-the-counter sugar-free fiber supplements. But there's more to it than fiber. Sometimes people don't drink enough water or don't eat enough fat. It may sound crazy, but if you're really focused on keeping fat calories down and carb calories down, even though you're getting an adequate amount of protein and some fresh green vegetables and those kinds of things, if you don't have enough fat in your diet, you can become constipated.

You may also want to look at exactly what protein sources you're using. Some people are relatively sensitive to the arachidonic acid found in red meat and egg yolks. If you look back at your diet diary and see that almost every day, almost every meal of protein is either red meat or egg yolks, it may be that arachidonic acid is making you constipated. Try backing away from those foods a little and eat fresh fish if you can get it— particularly coldwater fish like salmon, sardines, or mackerel that are high in EPA fish oil.

Oddly enough, just as many people probably complain to us about diarrhea as others do about constipation. In our experience, it's just as common. Either way, we usually find that it starts a few days into the program and resolves as the program goes along. Bowel changes are just one of those things that come about with any change in the diet. Don't worry about the constipation or diarrhea unless it continues. If it does, you need to see your doctor to make sure that some other reason isn't causing it.

I've been following the plan with great results but have noticed that my hair seems to be falling out. Is this due to the diet?

Any major physical stress or insult, such as surgery, high fever, severe trauma, or pregnancy can cause some of the hair follicles to enter a dormant state. The same thing happens to some people when they follow an unhealthy diet, such as a high-carbohydrate, low-protein one. A dormant hair shaft stops growing. When the insult passes—in the case of diet, once people begin to follow a healthier plan, such as a richer-protein, lower-carb diet—the hair follicles reactivate and begin to grow a new hair shaft, which forces the old dead hair out. A brand new healthy hair is replacing the old, dead hair. This kind of hair loss usually begins a couple of months after a dietary change for the better. If you're concerned, check with a dermatologist who can verify that tiny new healthy hairs are now coming in to replace those lost.

After being on the plan, I noticed that my nails are starting to crack and peel. Can you explain why this is happening?

Usually, nails that crack and peel can be the result of a nutrient excess or deficiency. Increased levels of iron or even excess vitamin A can cause this problem. Check to see that you are not taking in excess amounts of these nutrients. Taking vitamin A as beta-carotene may be a safer and more controlled way for you to supplement this vitamin. If you're eating plenty of meats, you shouldn't need to take extra iron supplementation.

I've heard that eating larger amounts of meat and shellfish can cause elevated uric acid levels, and I have a history of gout. Will this diet cause a gout episode?

Increased levels of uric acid are associated with insulin resistance, which results from a high intake of sugars and starchy foods. Most people with gout have a problem with either underexcretion of uric acid from the kidneys or overproduction of it due to specific enzyme defects.

On a high-carb diet that keeps insulin levels high, uric acid gets stored in the tissues and appears at high levels in the blood. The low-carb diet is a powerful force that causes a drop in insulin and uric acid levels. As these elevated levels begin to drop from decreased carbohydrate intake, the uric acid becomes mobilized and can crystallize within the joints, causing an attack of gout. The diet didn't cause the gout; it just worked to quickly drop high uric acid levels. It's the rapid fall in uric acid that prompts the attack. The same thing would occur if you were to begin taking prescription medications to reduce uric acid when the levels were very high.

If you know you're at risk for gout—you've had an attack in the past or it runs strongly in your family—ask a physician to check blood work to determine your uric acid levels. If they're very high, your doctor can prescribe medication to prevent the attack as you start the diet. Then the diet, like medication to lower uric acid, will quickly do its job to reduce the levels in your blood, and you'll no longer be at risk for future attacks as long as you follow the diet. At that point, your doctor can discontinue the preventive medication.

In addition, it's important for you to drink plenty of fluids, to supplement with magnesium, and not to go on and off the plan.

I have a history of kidney stones. Will following the plan cause them to become worse?

Some people's bodies form kidney stones more easily than others do. Changing to a low-carb, adequate-protein diet will not cause stone formation. What may happen with some individuals is that once their insulin levels start to drop due to a lower intake of carbohydrates, the diuretic effect will cause a stone that is already present to move. Movement of the stone causes the pain. Taking in plenty of water and magnesium, as well as lots of low-sugar fruits and green leafy veggies, will help to prevent the problem. We also suggest that you do not regularly take any extra calcium supplements, since this is what most stones are formed from.

I've been on the plan for a while and feel better than I ever have. I've lost weight, my blood pressure is down, and my sugar levels are now normal. My most recent lab tests show that my cholesterol and LDL went up. Am I doing something wrong?

First of all, be aware that you're not doing anything wrong. The most consistent finding after people go on our program is that triglycerides drop and HDL, the good cholesterol, increases. This indicates that your insulin levels have dropped and you have stopped converting excess amounts of sugar into fats as triglycerides. Cholesterol is a number that is composed of both good and bad fractions; therefore, we don't tend to track it nearly as closely as we do the more specific levels of HDL, triglycerides, and LDL. LDL cholesterol is made up of different-sized particles that vary from person to person.

Depending on the type of particles that predominate, one is said to have either pattern A or pattern B. With pattern A, the LDL is light, fluffy, and relatively large. This pattern is actually thought to be beneficial. With pattern B, the particles are heavy, dense, and relatively small. This pattern is thought to be detrimental. Pattern B is a partial consequence of excessively elevated triglycerides. When triglycerides go down on Protein Power or any low-carb diet, a phenomenon called the "beta shift" occurs where LDL is transformed into pattern A. So, paradoxically, even though the level of LDL appears to increase, the type of LDL that is being formed is usually much more beneficial. Unfortunately, the lab testing that is necessary to determine your levels of LDL "A" and LDL

"B" is not yet widely available. While we cannot be 100 percent certain that this is what happened in your case, the research strongly supports this view.

The most important thing is to look at the overall picture. In our experience, the triglyceride/HDL ratio is one of the best measurements of risk for heart disease. An upper limit of 5 is considered desirable, with anything over that indicating an increased risk. On our plan, most people will reach a ratio of 2 or less—a very healthy measurement indeed. Some steps to help bring down your cholesterol and LDL levels are to stay on the plan (some people panic and feel that the plan is causing the opposite effect); take "no-flush" niacin, 1,000 to 1,500 mg per day; increase your fiber intake with perhaps psyllium seed powder, 1 to 2 tablespoons mixed in water per day; and concern yourself with the quality of the fats you eat. Add a good-quality fish oil, eat more coldwater fish, avoid excessive saturated fats from processed meats, and cut out all transfats from vegetable oils, shortening, fried foods, and margarine.

I have been using Ketostix strips to monitor my ketone production, and initially, they were purple, but lately there is no indication of ketone production. What am I doing wrong?

We've never really focused on ketone production or monitoring ketone levels. However, many people do, and they like to see the stick turn purple as evidence of fat burning. As you've seen, it can be a real motivator when it's purple, but a real downer when it's not. Here's what happened.

On a high-carbohydrate diet, the body predominant uses sugar as its fuel source. When you convert to a low-carbohydrate diet, sugar isn't as available, so the body is forced to use fat as its main energy source. Initially, the enzymes that are needed for fat metabolism are not as efficient and available. One of the by-products of fat metabolism is the production of ketones (nothing more than partially burned fat), which is why you see purple on your Ketostix strip. As you continue on a low-carb diet, your body will become much more efficient at fat metabolism and will make use of the ketones as fuel for energy, burning them up completely. At that point, you won't see the evidence of so many ketones on your Ketostix strip. This doesn't mean that you aren't burning fat as your fuel source, but rather, that the body has just become efficient at using it fully. It's our opinion that the Ketostix approach is most helpful during the early stages of converting to a low-carb diet, because it does give you a visual report card that you're doing something.

Questions about Plateaus or Lack of Results

I have hit a plateau. What can I do to get things going again?

Everyone will plateau at some point on any diet—even on a low-carb diet. The body gets accustomed to its present demands and becomes very efficient at its job, therefore requiring fewer calories to do the same amount of work. Plateaus can last for different lengths of time, but after about three weeks, if you don't see results, you need to make some changes. It's time to fine-tune the diet for continued success.

First, if you've been lax about keeping your daily journal, you need to again start writing down everything you eat and drink for the next two weeks. This can take time and energy, but it's the best tool for understanding where the problem lies.

Potential problems areas are

1. You have unconsciously increased your carbohydrates too much— drop your carbs back down to the small serving level at three meals and one snack. Go back to the Low-Carb Boot Camp meal plans and follow them to the letter, or dust off your original corrective level low-carb diet and follow it faithfully. Focus on the portion size of all foods, and be sure to count all the extra carbs in foods such as nuts, cottage cheese, and dressings.

2. You might be eating either too much protein (excess calories) or not enough to fuel your metabolism. Go back to the Protein Requirements chart in appendix A and reassess your protein needs; don't exceed this portion size at meals or snacks, but always try to at least meet it.

3. You may be eating too many fat calories. Although healthful fats are acceptable on the plan and we don't normally recommend that you count the total grams of fat, you may be eating too many of them and, hence, ingesting too many calories. Nuts, nut butters, and cheese are the three top offenders, but don't forget that seeds, olives, oils, butter, and fatty protein choices such as bacon, sausage, and salami are all high in calories for the nutrition they

provide and are potential problem foods. Cut back on your intake of these foods. If you're a small person, you may not be able to tolerate as many calories as you're eating. You have to create a deficit to lose fat, and if you take in more calories than you burn, you won't lose weight. Make minor adjustments by limiting nuts to 1-ounce portions, selecting leaner cuts of meat, opting for low-fat dairy products, and adding more fish. If you're a big coffee drinker and you put cream in your coffee, you might try drinking fewer cups or switching to herbal tea throughout the day.

Try not to focus on weight loss as much. Instead, focus more on fat loss. After all, 6 pounds of fat take up a gallon of space—visualize those plastic gallon milk jugs dropping away one by one. Because fat takes up a lot of space, even a small weight change can translate into dramatic size changes. Remember that lean body mass weighs more than fat. If you get on the scale and you've lost 3 pounds of fat in a week but you've gained 3 pounds of muscle, you won't see any weight difference. But you are making progress! In actuality, you've recomposed your body. You're slimmer; it's just not reflected on the scale. One way to check that out is at the very beginning of your plan, choose one article of clothing—a pair of jeans or a fitted skirt—and use that article of clothing as your benchmark. If it's too tight when you begin, once a week, every week, try to put that piece of clothing on. Some weeks your progress may not show up on the scale, but it will show in the way your clothing fits.

Something else to be aware of is that you may have gained muscle. If you start an exercise program—especially if it's a weight-resistance program—you're going to build some muscle. So you may be going along losing weight and then, boom, suddenly stop. What may be happening is that you're exchanging body fat weight for lean muscle weight. Just keep in mind that this is a good thing. When you swap a pound of fat for a pound of muscle, it's always good. Muscle is metabolically active lean tissue; it uses more calories than fat does. And every pound of lean muscle you build is that many more calories you burn in a day.

I've been on the plan for a few weeks but haven't seen any results. Why?
The first thing to do if you're not seeing any progress is to check your measurements. It's probable that you're losing size even if the scale isn't

moving. Next, check your food portion sizes. It's especially important not to overdo it with cheeses, nuts, or nut butters, because the fat and calorie content is so high. In our years in practice, if someone was not making progress, these particular foods were almost always the main culprits. However, with the explosion of low-carb products on the market, most of them plastered with labels often erroneously trumpeting "0, 1, or 2 net carbs," there are now many more potential diet-sabotaging candidates. These products give lots of room for too many carb-free calories. The simple fact is that you must create a calorie deficit to lose weight; in other words, calories taken in have to be less than calories going out, even if you're taking in mainly protein and healthful fats. There is even an outside possibility that you could be exceeding your protein requirement by too much at each meal. Though we always say that the protein requirement is a minimum and not a maximum, if you do exceed it by a wide margin every day, you may have trouble getting weight reduction results.

Keep a journal of every bite of food and drink you put in your mouth. Although you must be meticulous about your portions, be certain that you take in at least your minimum protein requirement. You need protein to support your lean mass, which fuels your metabolic rate, but don't go overboard. Keep meticulous count of your carbohydrate intake. There are a lot of hidden carbs and many calories in foods such as condiments, nuts, dairy products, and low-carb packaged foods. Read your labels!

Is it okay to eat foods that contain artificial sweeteners?

Yes, but you want to be careful when choosing which artificial sweetener to use, and you should use them only in moderation. Based on recent information that suggests that aspartame (NutraSweet, Equal) may be harmful to brain cells, we recommend that you avoid it. Saccharin, stevia, acesulfame (marketed as SweetOne), and Splenda (sucralose) are better choices.

Another reason to avoid artificial sweeteners is that the intense sweet taste can actually trick your body and stimulate the release of insulin. In turn, your blood sugar will drop and you may experience hunger. So in the long run, artificial sweeteners may cause you to overeat when otherwise you would not.

Quick Start Plan to Help Break a Plateau

If you have derailed on the plan and want to get back on track in a hurry, try cutting carbs and calories for a week. Drink a protein powder shake for two meals each day, along with one dinner meal from the Low-Carb Boot Camp, to help to kick-start your progress. Choose a low-carb protein powder, mix with water and a few frozen strawberries or raspberries, ice cubes, and about 1 ounce of half and half, and you'll have a delicious, nutritious, and filling meal. Be sure to take your potassium and magnesium supplements, about 200 to 600 mg of magnesium and 200 to 400 mg of potassium each day. Drink a minimum of 2 quarts of water a day and *exercise!*

Supplements That Complement the Protein Power Diet

We recommend that you take a good overall multiple vitamin and mineral supplement that does not contain iron. The reason that we don't recommend additional iron through supplementation is that even though iron is essential to the body, in excess it becomes an oxidant and can cause damage to organs such as the heart, liver, thyroid gland, pancreas, and others. If you're interested in learning more about the dangers of excess iron, you'll find an entire chapter on the subject in our book *The Protein Power LifePlan.*

Magnesium: An essential mineral, magnesium is involved in over 300 metabolic processes. It has been called nature's calcium channel blocker, and as such is essential for people with hypertension. It is also indicated for health conditions such as cardiac arrhythmias, diabetes mellitus, osteoporosis, alcoholism, migraines, premenstrual syndrome, and vascular disease, to mention a few. Magnesium levels are depleted through stress, which is present in everyone's life. In excessive doses, magnesium can cause diarrhea; you're probably familiar with it as the milk-of-magnesia effect. Recommended dosage: 200 to 600 mg per day or up to bowel tolerance.

Potassium: An electrolyte important in the transmission of nerve impulses; contraction of cardiac, skeletal, and smooth muscles; production of energy; and maintenance of blood pressure, as well as other important functions. The main cause of potassium depletion is excessive loss through the kidneys or the gastrointestinal tract. Because a low-carb corrective diet initially causes loss of excess fluids, as well as of electrolytes (magnesium, potassium, sodium), it's essential to take potassium supplements, especially during the early phases of the plan. Signs of potassium deficiency include muscle weakness, fatigue, listlessness, heart palpitations or flutters, and loss of appetite. Recommended dosage is 200 to 400 mg or more per day.

Chromium polynicotinate: Chromium is an essential trace mineral that plays a key role in normal carbohydrate metabolism. It helps to regulate glucose levels and lower cholesterol levels. It is claimed to be helpful for people with diabetes. It can boost athletic performance, it builds muscle, and it promotes weight loss. Average recommended dosages range from 200 mcg (note *micro*grams here) per day to a total of 800 mcg per day.

Alpha Lipoic Acid: Thioctic acid, also known as alpha lipoic acid, is a potent fat- and water-soluble antioxidant. It is vital to the energy-producing reactions in the body. In Germany, it is an approved drug for the treatment of nerve disorders (numbness, tingling) from disease conditions such as diabetes and alcoholism. It is also useful against oxidative stress, arteriosclerosis, and various radiologic and chemical toxins. It may lower blood glucose levels, so people with diabetes who take it need to monitor their blood sugar levels closely. Recommended dosages range from 300 to 600 mg or more daily, depending on the condition being treated.

Coenzyme Q10: A member of the ubiquinone family, Co Q10 is a water-insoluble substance involved in electron transport and energy production. Supplementation may protect the heart, brain, and nervous system, and the delicate fats in the cell membranes of all the tissues in the body. It is best absorbed in an oil-based form or with a meal containing fat. Absorption on an empty stomach is poor. Levels of the body's natural production of Co Q10 fall in people taking the statin drugs to lower blood cholesterol. The usual recommended dosage ranges from 100 to 200 mg per day, taken with food, however individuals taking statin drugs should take at least 300 mg of supplemental Co Q10 daily.

Vitamin E: Vitamin E, or alpha tocopherol, is a fat-soluble vitamin. It has antioxidant activities; thins the blood; protects the brain, nerves, and skin; and helps to prevent arteriosclerosis and the formation of blood clots, just to mention a few of its important activities. It also appears to be protective against cardiovascular disease and some forms of cancer. Recommended dosages range from 400 to 1,000 mg per day.

Pentabosol: Our newest all-natural weight-loss supplement designed to work with a low-carb diet. It is a combination of five natural ingredients, designed to metabolically increase the fat-metabolism processes. For further information, please visit www.pentabosol.com.

Other Supplemental Nutrients: We have used numerous other supplements in our practice that help to control blood sugar levels and improve fat metabolism, act as antioxidants, and help with metabolism in general. Some of these include niacinamide for lowering cholesterol levels, pantothenic acid (vitamin B_5) for supporting the stress response, zinc for prostate health and to support immunity, bilberry for eye health, L-carnitine for fat metabolism, L-glutamine for blood-sugar regulation and gut healing, and vanadyl sulfate for insulin support and carbohydrate metabolism. For further information regarding the supplements we recommend, visit our Web site www.proteinpower.com.

Specific Issues about Following a Low-Carbohydrate Diet

Is there anyone who should avoid a low-carbohydrate diet?

People with documented kidney disease (by that, we mean individuals with documented reduced renal function) need to be more careful following a higher-protein diet. Managing kidney disease requires being very careful about all intake: food, fluid, vitamins, and minerals. People who suffer from reduced kidney function should not exceed their minimum protein intake and may do better dividing it into five or six small meals and snacks. If you have kidney disease, please work with your doctor to monitor your kidney function through lab testing.

How will the diet affect women's menstrual cycles or someone on estrogen replacement therapy?

Insulin is a powerful hormone with many responsibilities, one of them being to promote the storage of calories as fat. Estrogen is normally stored in body fat, where one of the steps in its metabolism occurs. The more body fat you have, the more estrogen can be stored there. When levels of insulin fall with the decrease in carbohydrates, your body begins to unpack the fat from storage. Any substance stored in the fat will, of course, also be brought out into the blood as the fat is mobilized and burned. So during fat loss, estrogen levels may become unbalanced, possibly causing a disruption in menstrual cycles. Some women may notice spotting or break-through bleeding at midcycle, or their flow may become lighter or heavier. We recommend being patient, continuing on the plan, and within two to three cycles, the hormone levels should come back into balance. If the symptoms persist, we recommend seeing your gynecologist to be sure something else isn't the cause of the menstrual change.

During menopause, levels of reproductive hormones begin to decline with a shift toward catabolism (bone and muscle wasting). Estrogen replacement alone or with Provera can promote fluid retention and fat gain—and as recent studies have shown, can increase the risk for heart disease and cancer. When necessary, we recommend the use of natural estrogen and progesterone compounds, applied topically. Ask your doctor about changing from synthetic estrogen and progestin (Premarin/Provera) to a natural formulation, and this may help speed your fat loss and normalize your fluid retention problems.

In women who have undergone hysterectomy and ovarian removal, some natural estrogen may be necessary, but in women who still have functioning ovaries, natural progesterone by itself may be a better option. Eating a low-carb diet, rich in good-quality fats and cholesterol, will promote higher levels of the "mother" hormones from which reproductive hormones must be made after the ovaries begin to slow down or cease production. The diet also provides a better magnesium-to-calcium balance, which, along with the natural estrogen and progesterone, will keep bones strong and ward off osteoporosis.

Can you follow a low-carb diet at all while you're pregnant or nursing?

Pregnancy and nursing place an increased demand on the mother for both calories and protein. It is not safe to undertake a reduced-calorie intervention during these times. You'll also need more protein than before—up your intake to the next-larger protein serving size than your height and weight would suggest. For instance, if the Protein Requirements chart suggests a small serving of protein for your height and weight, eat a medium serving size. That said, a sensible low-carb *maintenance level* diet is actually a very healthy nutritional structure for women during pregnancy and afterward, offering plenty of lean protein, dairy products, fresh colorful vegetables and fruits, no refined sugar, and minimal wheat, corn, or potato starch. As long as you have normal, healthy kidneys, it's a great nutritional regimen.

Add the extra calories that are necessary to maintain weight during these special conditions (pregnancy and lactation) as lean protein, dairy, or good-quality fats, and keep the carbohydrates at the moderate-to-large-serving level, choosing from fresh fruits, green leafy and colorful vegetables, and beans as much as possible.

Remember, you can have more protein and more good fat, but keep the carbohydrates fixed near this maintenance level. And remember, too, to check any nutritional changes with your obstetrician before you make them.

Is this program safe for a child?

Normal-weight children can follow the basic guidelines of the plan—selecting from all the foods available to you—but without restriction on quantity. We don't recommend that children follow a reduced-calorie diet unless they are tremendously overweight—and then only under the advice and care of a physician. An excessively overweight child or teen should be evaluated by an endocrine specialist to be certain there aren't any hormonal disturbances or even benign pituitary gland tumors contributing to the weight problem. If there are no contributing problems, the child could follow the general transition or maintenance level guidelines of the plan.

Don't make an issue of your children's weight or try to put severe restrictions on the foods they eat—as long as they're good foods, not junk. Those tactics will usually prove counterproductive. Even if children are somewhat overweight, it's a better idea to offer them a healthy diet at home, engage them in plenty of physical exercise with their families, and let the children grow into the weight over time. Unlike adults, kids are still growing in the upward direction, and ultimately, if their weight doesn't increase, but their height does, they'll slim down. Be patient.

Encourage your children to consume a protein-based food at each meal—eggs, meat, fish, poultry, cheese, or dairy. Growing children (and, interestingly enough, the elderly) need more protein per pound of lean body weight than young or middle-aged adults do.

Encourage your kids to make healthy choices of wholesome carbohydrates from fruits, vegetables, beans, rice, oats, and whole grains. They should limit or avoid sweets, excess refined starches, and empty calories from sweetened cereals. Don't keep these items in your home. We also advise children to drink plenty of fresh water, milk, and some fruit juice, but to limit sodas and fruit drink beverages, which are nothing but fruit-flavored sugar water. Set a positive example for your children to follow, by making good-quality nutritious foods available to them at home for meals and snacks. These nutritional rules apply to both overweight kids and normal weight ones.

Is this program safe for vegetarians?

As a vegetarian, you may find it difficult but not impossible to follow a lower-carbohydrate diet. Because you're limited in your protein choices, you have to be creative to promote variety in your diet. Protein for vegans will come primarily from soy-based products such as tofu, TVP, soybeans, and nuts. Ovo-lacto vegetarians will add protein from eggs and dairy products. A few less-stringent vegetarians will consume fish, which is a wonderful complete healthy protein. To these protein sources, all vegetarians will add a variety of fibrous, low-starch vegetables, low-sugar fruits, and healthy fat sources, such as olives, avocado, fish oil, and flax seeds or flaxseed oil.

Many of the foods that traditional vegetarians have customarily eaten for protein—dried beans, other legumes, and grain products—are laden with too many carbohydrates to make them useful on a corrective level low-carb diet. Even though these foods do contain some protein, the carb load is too high to use them as your sole protein source. Carnitine and extra B vitamins, particularly B_{12}, are essential for vegetarians who don't eat eggs or dairy products.

How does this diet affect endurance athletes?

Quite well, once you've adapted to using fat as your main fuel for exercise, a process that may take a week or two. If you make a switch to low carb and immediately try to bike or run, you'll probably think that your performance suffers, but there's an explanation for this phenomenon, and it's transient. Here's what happens. Carbohydrate restriction causes a slight depletion of the glycogen stores. For a few days this condition may cause slight fatigue and a feeling of being out of gas, but it is the slightly glycogen-depleted state that encourages the body to turn to fat as the preferred metabolic fuel for muscle. Once that switch to using fat as fuel occurs, endurance improves again and will ultimately exceed the carb-fueled level, because even in a lean person, there's a lot more fat than glycogen to draw from. In studies done at the Naval Health Research Center in San Diego, Captain Charles Gray has shown that after adapting to the low-carb state, naval recruits not only equaled their previous endurance level, they surpassed it. Nowadays, athletes who do well in endurance events tend to load up on fats more than they do on carbohydrates, because all the recent studies show that fat loading promotes better athletic endurance.

What's wrong with carb loading before athletic events?

When you're on a higher-carbohydrate diet, the whole premise of carb loading is that you're trying to stuff a lot of glycogen into your glycogen stores so that you can run on it. But no matter how full you stuff them, they can get only so full. A full tank of glycogen lasts only a couple of hours. You can't run on glycogen for longer than that, so athletes hit the wall; they run out of steam and have to switch over to burning fat. If they started burning fat right at the beginning, they'd do much better. The other problem with carb loading is that becoming carbohydrate-adapted often means that your insulin levels increase. And in the face of elevated insulin levels, you can't easily access the fat stored in your fat cells. The fat in your fat cells is your most important and most potent source of energy in any kind of endurance event. Remember, you get 9 calories of energy from 1 gram of fat versus 4 calories of energy from 1 gram of carbohydrate. No matter how well somebody's doing athletically, on a high-protein, lower-carb, higher-fat plan, he or she could probably do better, once allowed to adapt.

I'm a bodybuilder, training for a competition. How do I incorporate a low-carb diet into my routine?

A lower-carb diet is the perfect plan for a bodybuilder. It's very important to know what your lean mass weighs, because your maintenance protein intake will be based on that number of pounds times your activity level. For most builders, the number usually comes in somewhere around 1 to 1.2 grams of protein per pound of lean mass per day. Because your protein intake may get as high as 300 to 400 grams of protein per day, it's important to eat small amounts about every one to three hours. Your carbohydrate intake will be less than half of your protein intake, consisting mainly of the fibrous vegetables and a few fruits. Keep your fat intake to healthy choices and at a moderate level, in order to force your body to burn stored fat as its energy source. This is what will give you that cut, lean appearance. Drink a half-gallon of water a day and replace those electrolytes.

Should I exercise on this plan?

An exercise program is as important to fitness and health as a sound low-carb diet is. Many people, for different reasons, are unable to exercise, so we always stress the importance of the diet first. Our stance on exercise is that we feel weight-resistance training will give you more bang for your buck, not only from a time and financial investment but also from a health investment. Our book *The Slow Burn Fitness Revolution,* coauthored with fitness expert Fred Hahn, offers the latest cutting-edge information on what we feel is the ideal exercise program. Take the time to read the book and engage in the workout routines, whether at home or at the gym. We recommend that you make it an integral part of your low-carb lifestyle.

While strength training is clearly the winner in building muscle, strong bones, and strength, aerobic exercise and plain old recreation are also beneficial to augment your program. If you love to run, walk, bike, swim, or dance, get out there and do it. If you enjoy doing yoga, by all means, keep at it. If you love a rousing tennis match, go for it. Join your friends for a pick-up basketball or touch football game in the park. Remember, calories do count and the rule is: you have to expend more calories than you take in in order to lose pounds. Do what you enjoy!

I'm happy with my weight but would like to follow the diet for health reasons. How do I keep from losing weight and yet follow a low-carb diet?

It's important for everyone to start at a lower-carb amount to convert the body into primarily fat-burning metabolism. Calculate your protein requirements and be compliant with taking in at least that amount. Start at a small serving of carbohydrates at each of your three meals and one snack. In order to maintain your current weight as you cut carbs to resolve other health problems (cholesterol, triglycerides, blood sugar elevation, chronic reflux), you'll need to eat more calories from foods such as nuts, nut butters, seeds, olives, and cheese, which contain few carbs but lots of healthy fats. To give you an idea of how much you'll need to eat, remember that each ounce of nuts or cheese contains about 100 calories. Each tablespoon of butter, oil, or peanut butter contains about the same number. And a pound of fat loss corresponds with about 3,500 calories of deficit, which means that if you're losing a pound a week, you'll need to increase your daily caloric intake of calorie-dense low-carb foods by about 500 calories a day. Once you've corrected your health issues, you can move to transition and then to maintenance, where you won't have to spend so much time snacking on these calorie-dense foods.

Common Myths about Low-Carb Dieting

Can high-protein, low-carbohydrate diets damage your kidneys?

Not as long as you start out with normal kidney function. There are several key studies that lay this myth to rest. One study was done in Israel a few years ago. It compared people who ate lots of protein to people who had been vegetarians for an average of about thirteen years and who ate minimal amounts of protein. The only protein they consumed was vegetable protein. Researchers did careful cross matching, so that they had a near-perfect match in terms of age and sex in the two groups. When they compared the normal decline in kidney function that naturally occurs in people as they age, the researchers found no difference between the heavy-protein eaters and the low-protein eaters.

There have also been several studies out of Germany from a group of researchers who studied bodybuilders, who tend to eat lots of protein to build muscle. Those researchers discovered that higher-protein diets do not cause kidney deterioration but instead enhance kidney function. The protein actually makes the kidneys function more efficiently.

The only time that high-protein diets can affect kidney function is if you have impaired kidney function to begin with. If you do have a serious kidney problem—and most people who have one know they do—it doesn't mean you shouldn't eat any protein. If you don't eat protein, you'll become protein-malnourished. What it does mean is that you have to be very careful to eat only the minimum amount allowed. You can't go over it. But for the vast majority of us who have normal kidney function, eating more protein doesn't hurt our kidneys at all.

Do diets that are higher in protein cause a loss of calcium and weaken our bones? Will it make me prone to osteoporosis?

The theory behind this idea is that when you eat protein, it's broken down into substances that are a little bit acidic. Supposedly, if there's nothing alkaline to balance it, this more-acidic blood somehow leaches the calcium out of the bones, and it can end up giving us osteoporosis at a later date.

All of that sounds logical, but in fact it just doesn't happen, except in people who follow extremely low-carb diets devoid of fruits and vegetables for many years. This theory has been studied extensively over long periods of time. What researchers have found is that when people eat a lot of protein, especially meat protein, along with a balance of fresh fruits and vegetables or some other alkaline source to balance the acid load (such as alkaline drinking water), they don't have any increase in urinary calcium. In other words, they're not leaching the calcium out of their bones and losing it in their urine, as the theory would imply.

And when we look at the skeletal remains of hunters and gatherers who ate two to three times the amount of protein recommended as safe for us today, we find that their bones are 17 percent more dense than ours given that the comparison is done between individuals of the same height and gender.

Finally, there's another part of the bone-loss story that you may not have heard: grains and cheese are acidic, too. A grain-based diet that isn't balanced by alkaline sources from fresh fruits, green leafies, and colorful veggies or alkaline water will be just as damaging to bones as a pure meat diet. The worst diet of all for bone loss would be a diet high in meat, cheese, and grain—that describes the typical All-American cheeseburger. Is it any wonder that osteoporosis is on the rise? Wrap that burger in a big lettuce leaf, enjoy a garden salad of fresh veggies and lettuce, and you won't need to worry about your bones.

Don't vegetarian diets help people lose weight and cure diseases like cancer?

On any calorie-restrictive diet, your insulin level will fall and you'll lose some weight. Many people who follow a vegetarian lifestyle lose tremendous amounts of weight. It's important to remember, however, that losing weight is not the same as losing fat. On a diet that is deficient in protein, as much as 50 percent of the weight lost may be from the lean body, not the fat mass. Weight is weight, and it will certainly show up as a loss on the scale, but losing muscle is ultimately counterproductive, since it is the lean mass that determines metabolic rate. The more you lose from this part of you, the lower your metabolic rate will become.

No evidence suggests that vegetarian diets cure cancer. The higher levels of phytochemicals from fresh colorful vegetables may help to prevent some cancers, but a diet that's high in good-quality lean meat will stimulate the immune system even more. And a diet high in both lean meats and lots of colorful fruits and vegetables is even better. A sensible low-carb diet provides multiple benefits: it helps you to lose body fat instead of lean mass; it provides quality protein to support your immune system; and it's rich in green and colorful veggies and fruits that provide cancer-fighting phytochemicals to boot!

Final Words of Advice

Which foods should I avoid when starting a lower-carbohydrate diet?

The obvious ones are the sweet treats, such as traditionally prepared cakes, pies, cookies, candy, and ice cream, as well as fruit juices, sweeter fruits (such as bananas, papayas, raisins, dates, figs, mangos, and dried fruits), potatoes, sweet potatoes, rice, pasta, fried foods, chips, crackers, breads, muffins, bagels, soda pop, ketchup, BBQ sauce, excess coffee, and alcohol. Once you reach your goal, small portions of these foods can be added on a rotational basis. And don't forget that many lower-carb versions of these treats are becoming available and that you can make many of them using recipes you'll find in our *Low-Carb Comfort Food Cookbook,* available at bookstores everywhere or online.

What are the best choices for salad dressings?

Creamy dressings made from cream cheese, sour cream, or cottage cheese with seasonings; cheese-based dressings such as blue cheese and Roquefort; ranch; traditional vinaigrettes; simple vinegar and oil; or just lemon juice are acceptable. You'll find many delicious low-carb dressing recipes in *The Low-Carb Comfort Food Cookbook* and others, and many tasty lower-carbohydrate dressings are becoming available at grocery and health food stores.

How important is water in my diet?

Very! In general, we recommend at least 6 to 8 cups of water a day—that's about 2 quarts of water—but people's needs differ, based on their body size and shape. To calculate your body's water intake needs, multiply your weight by .69 for the number of ounces, then divide that number by 8 for the total number of glasses of water needed each day. Remember that although your best choice is good fresh water, caffeine-free coffees, teas, and herbal teas also count as water.

What should I do if I get hungry between meals?

If you feel hungry, eat some form of protein—leftover steak or chicken, deli meat, or an ounce or two of cheese. Raw or dry roasted nuts or seeds work, too. These kinds of snacks will keep your blood sugar stable and take longer to digest than carbs do, keeping you from experiencing carbohydrate yo-yo cravings. A protein shake is also a great snack for in-between meal hunger.

What are protein shakes or smoothies, and how do I incorporate them into my diet?

A protein shake or a smoothie is made from a quality low-carb protein powder that contains no more than 2 to 3 grams of carbohydrate per serving. Mixing the powder with only water will provide the shake with the fewest carbohydrates but also the blandest taste. Frozen berries or melon add flavor without too many carbs or calories. Ice cubes will create a thicker shake. Adding light cream, nut butters, or coconut milk can add richness and variety, but they do add calories and some carbs. A protein shake can be used as a meal or a snack.

If I know I will be eating dessert, how do I calculate it into my diet?

The ideal time to eat sweet treats is earlier in the day, when your insulin sensitivity is highest. Earlier also gives you time to burn it off through daily activities. However, if a special occasion arises in the evening and you know you'll be offered a dessert that you can't (or don't want to) avoid, lower your carbohydrate intake for the entire day, including the meal that you will follow with the dessert. We know this violates the you-can't-save-up-your-carbs rule, but it's okay to do it for a special occasion. Always eat dessert with your meal, never alone. Plan the times you will be eating dessert. This helps to keep you on target and allows you to make appropriate adjustments to your carbohydrate intake that day. Always get back on target immediately. Don't let eating dessert—even if it's unplanned—be an excuse to derail your diet.

What can I do to overcome cravings?

There can be a lot of reasons why you crave a given food. Maybe it's something you use to treat yourself when you feel low or to reward success. Maybe it's a comfort food your mom used to give you when you were sick. Maybe it's a cultural tradition, like a hot dog at the ball game. Your mind has set up these emotional or mental connections between events, feelings, and food. Once you're in maintenance, you may be able to enjoy these occasional indulgences. You can modify some of them in ways that will fit your new lifestyle, using low-carb ingredients and recipes you'll find in *The Low-Carb Comfort Food Cookbook* and from other sources, and still be able to enjoy them. But for now, it's best that you view these cravings as habits you're trying to break. Here are some strategies that may help.

- Anticipate the craving. If cravings set in at a particular time of the day, plan a healthy low-carb snack to eat at that time—preferably before the craving sets in. Eating a high-protein, higher-fat snack will fill you up and may take the craving away. An ounce of cheese or nuts, a handful of grapes, and a big glass of iced tea or water will often quiet the craving for sugary things. A craving for savory foods is easy to quell—have some leftover steak or a few pork rinds or nuts. That's one craving you can give in to.

- Substitute a desirable activity. If you always had a candy bar when you became frustrated at work, substitute a new activity. Try getting up from your desk and taking a walk. If you always stopped off for a bagel on your way to work, try another route that doesn't take you past the bagel shop. If your cravings hit at home, go outside and work in the yard, start a project in the workshop, take a shower, or paint your nails. Find another activity to take your mind off eating.

- Wait ten minutes. This strategy works well for smokers trying to quit, so it should work for you, too. If a craving strikes, tempting you to eat something you shouldn't, wait ten minutes. Make a deal with yourself that if you still crave it in ten minutes, you can have it. Most of the time you'll go off, get involved in something else, and forget all about it. Try this a couple of times, but if it doesn't work for you, abandon the strategy. Don't use the ten-minute rule as an excuse to eat more than you should.

- Start a new tradition. If you always have a hot dog at the ballpark, while you're in the corrective phase of your plan, try having just the naked dog without the bun. The taste is about the same and the carb cost much less. Dip the dog in mustard and dill pickle relish and enjoy.

    If you join your girlfriends for pastries at the local coffee shop in the afternoon, switch the agenda. Meet in the park for a walk and a talk, meet at the health club for a sauna, or go to a movie. If you always get popcorn at the movies, try smuggling in a zip-lock bag of buttered almonds instead and get a large soda water at the concession stand.

    If you always stop for beers with the boys on Thursdays after work, get together at the gym for a workout.

How do I stick to the plan while traveling?

When traveling, it can be challenging at best to comply with a low-carb regime. Now that you know how to eat, do your best by making the choices that will support your newfound lifestyle. Always have appropriate snacks available in case you have to skip a meal because of travel arrangements. Keep nuts, seeds, protein bars, jerky, or homemade low-carb cookies or crackers in reach. It's not unusual to find that you end up eating more carbohydrates when on the road—it happens to us, too—so don't get too stressed about it. Once you're back home and into a routine again, become refocused on the corrective phase of your plan to knock off any addition fluid or weight you've added. That way, you'll get back on track immediately. Always carry a water bottle with you. Drinking fluids will keep you feeling full and satisfied if there are too many hours between meals.

Eating Out

It's becoming increasingly easier to eat out and stay on your low-carb plan. Most restaurants are willing to make substitutions for the starchy vegetables and grains that they serve. Don't be afraid to ask for extra vegetables instead of the potato, rice, or pasta. Ask what soup bases are made of, and avoid the potato or starchy bases. A nice fibrous vegetable salad before your main entrée will set the stage. Basic entrees such as fish, poultry, or meat dishes and extra vegetables are perfect to help you comply with the plan. Tell your waiter not to bring bread or the dessert tray to the table. Stop eating when you feel full, and have the leftovers for lunch the next day. A glass of wine or a cocktail with your meal is also acceptable.

Fast food restaurants: If ordering a burger, a sandwich, or a hot dog, ask for it "protein style," wrapped in big crunchy lettuce leaves, or just take off the top bun. Half of a bun will give you about 10 grams of carb—your allotment if following the corrective phase. Add a salad to go with your burger, and it's still an acceptable low-carb meal.

Steak, chop, chicken, or seafood restaurants: Avoid bread, rolls, crackers, potatoes, rice, pasta, starchy vegetables, sugary desserts, sweet wines, and liquors. Begin with a protein appetizer, such as a shrimp cocktail or steamed mussels or clams. Then go for a big salad with an olive oil vinaigrette, ranch, or blue cheese dressing, or just lemon juice. Order your favorite cut of beef, lamb, pork chops, chicken breast, duck, fish, or seafood cooked any way you like except battered and fried.

Instead of potatoes, rice, or pasta, ask the waiter to substitute green or mixed veggies, slices of tomato, or another serving of salad. Select tea, coffee, or water to drink. If you like, enjoy a single glass of dry white or red wine or a low-carb light beer. Order fresh berries or melon for dessert, if in season. Or treat yourself to an after-dinner espresso or cappuccino.

Italian restaurants: Avoid bread, pasta dishes, and breaded dishes, such as eggplant or veal parmesan. Begin with a salad, an antipasto platter, sautéed calamari, steamed clams or mussels, or carpaccio. Order medallions of beef, roasted chicken, grilled beef, rabbit, fish, or seafood. Select a sauté of zucchini, squashes, peppers, or other veggies in place of pasta. Drink tea, coffee, water, one glass of dry red or white wine, or a single light beer. In season, enjoy misto bosco, fresh mixed berries, with whipped cream for dessert.

Pizza and sub restaurants: Avoid garlic bread, breadsticks, pizza crust, and more than half of a submarine or hoagie bun. Even half a bun may have a moderate serving of carbs all by itself. Start with a fresh green salad with ranch, blue cheese, or a vinaigrette dressing. Get pizza with all the toppings you love, then eat the tops and leave the crust. Order a sub with lots of meat, cheese, peppers, lettuce, tomato, and onion and eat the insides, leaving all or most of the bun. Drink tea, coffee, water, or a single glass of dry red or white wine or a single light beer.

Chinese, Vietnamese, and Thai restaurants: Avoid steamed or fried rice, noodles, wontons, breaded items, sweet and sour entrees, mooshoo pancakes, dim sum, egg rolls, and spring rolls. Begin with clear soup, avoiding the noodles, dumplings, or wontons. Ask for a green salad or some marinated vegetables. Choose grilled or stir-fried chicken, beef, pork, fish, or seafood along with veggies. There will usually be peppers, onions, mushrooms, water chestnuts, and bamboo shoots. There may be some cornstarch in the sauce, so beware of eating too much of it. Order a pot of hot black tea or green tea or just have water. If you're in transition or on maintenance, you could have a glass of dry wine or a light beer. In correction, the cornstarch and the veggies will take up most of your carb allotment. Read your fortune aloud and enjoy a laugh—then give the cookie away!

Japanese restaurants: Avoid tempura-fried foods; extra rice, especially sushi rice, which has added sugar to make it sticky; and hand rolls. In rolls, the rice is too difficult to separate from the fish, and you'll end up eating too much rice. Begin with miso soup and a green salad. Select any sort of fish or shellfish you prefer. Your best bet is to get them as sashimi, raw pieces of fish without rice. The second-best option is to order nigiri sushi, raw pieces of fish on a small ball of rice. Discard at least half of the rice from each piece of nigiri sushi. Enjoy green tea, iced tea, and water. If you've had sashimi, you should have enough carb room for a glass of dry wine or a light beer.

Burger restaurants: Avoid buns, breaded chicken or fish, French fries, and chips. Begin with a salad and good dressing. Order any single- or double-patty burger, grilled chicken, or grilled fish sandwich. Add cheese, bacon, or guacamole if you like. Have whatever accompaniments you desire—tomato, lettuce, onion, mushrooms, mustard, pickle—but watch the ketchup. Ask for two large green lettuce leaves to wrap your sandwich in. Some places (In-N-Out Burgers in California, for example) offer their burgers "protein style" done this way only on request. No bun, just two big crunchy leaves of iceberg lettuce wrapped around the meat. Drink iced tea, water, or a single light beer if you like. Some places offer fresh whole fruit—an orange, an apple, or a peach. Split a piece of fruit with a friend for dessert.

The Importance of Keeping a Journal

You'll see that we've included a 365-day Staying Power LifePlanner journal in *Staying Power* as appendix D. We've done so for a very specific reason. Studies have shown that when you're trying to make a lifestyle change—change the way you eat, engage in more exercise, give up old habits—your odds of success increase four times if you commit your goals to writing and keep a careful record of your progress. Your 365-day journal provides space for you to record what you eat at each meal or snack, what you drink, the supplements you take during the day, and the amount and kind of exercise you do. We've included space to plan your health and fitness goals for the week, a Protein Power tip, and a few words of inspiration and motivation from great writers and comedians throughout history.

We ask that you keep your journal with you, that you record each meal as you eat it, and that you use it as a tool to keep you on track toward reclaiming your health and fitness.

The layout is universal, going from January 1 to December 31, and no days or years are specified. Whatever day you start your new life plan, begin your journal record there. For instance, say you start your plan on

February 13; begin there, then when you get to the end of the year, go back to the start and use the front of the journal, filling in January 1 to February 12. Your 365 days would run from February 13 of one year to February 12 of the next.

You'll also notice that in the back of the journal, we've provided a blank health Progress Chart to help you track your progress. This way, it will be easy for you to see at a glance the trends of your cholesterol or triglycerides falling over time, your weight going down, and your measurements getting smaller. It will also help you to determine when you are nearing your goals and are ready to move ahead in your program, making the transition from corrective dieting to maintenance living.

Your journal is a success tool. Use it daily! We wish you good health and happiness for a lifetime.

Protein Requirements

Women

						Height							
Weight	5' or less	5'1"	5'2"	5'3"	5'4"	5'5"	5'6"	5'7"	5'8"	5'9"	5'10"	5'11"	6' and up
up to 100	S	S	S	S	S	S	S	S	S	M	M	M	M
105	S	S	S	S	S	S	S	M	M	M	M	M	M
110	S	S	S	M	M	M	M	M	M	M	M	M	M
115	M	M	M	M	M	M	M	M	M	M	M	M	M
120	M	M	M	M	M	M	M	M	M	M	M	M	M
125	M	M	M	M	M	M	M	M	M	M	M	M	M
130	M	M	M	M	M	M	M	M	M	M	M	M	M
135	M	M	M	M	M	M	M	M	M	M	M	M	L
140	M	M	M	M	M	M	M	M	M	M	M	L	L
145	M	M	M	M	M	M	M	M	M	M	M	L	L
150	M	M	M	M	M	M	M	M	L	L	L	L	L
155	M	M	M	M	M	M	L	L	L	L	L	L	L
160	M	M	M	M	M	L	L	L	L	L	L	L	L
165	M	M	M	M	L	L	L	L	L	L	L	L	L
170	M	M	M	L	L	L	L	L	L	L	L	L	L
175	M	M	L	L	L	L	L	L	L	L	L	L	L
180	L	L	L	L	L	L	L	L	L	L	L	L	L
185	L	L	L	L	L	L	L	L	L	L	L	L	L
190	L	L	L	L	L	L	L	L	L	L	L	L	L
195	L	L	L	L	L	L	L	L	L	L	L	L	L
200	L	L	L	L	L	L	L	L	L	L	L	L	L
205	L	L	L	L	L	L	L	L	L	L	L	L	L
210	L	L	L	L	L	L	L	L	L	X	X	L	L
215	L	L	L	L	L	L	L	L	X	X	X	X	X
220	L	L	L	L	L	L	L	X	X	X	X	X	X
225	L	L	L	L	L	L	X	X	X	X	X	X	X
230	L	L	L	L	L	X	X	X	X	X	X	X	X
235	L	L	L	L	L	X	X	X	X	X	X	X	X
240	L	L	L	X	X	X	X	X	X	X	X	X	X
245	L	L	X	X	X	X	X	X	X	X	X	X	X
250	X	L	X	X	X	X	X	X	X	X	X	X	X
255	X	X	X	X	X	X	X	X	X	X	X	X	X
260	X	X	X	X	X	X	X	X	X	X	X	X	X
265	X	X	X	X	X	X	X	X	X	X	X	X	X
270	X	X	X	X	X	X	X	X	X	X	X	X	X
275	X	X	X	X	X	X	X	X	X	X	X	X	X
280	X	X	X	X	X	X	X	X	X	X	X	X	X
285	X	X	X	X	X	X	X	X	X	X	X	X	X
290	X	X	X	X	X	X	X	X	X	X	X	X	X
295	X	X	X	X	X	X	X	X	X	X	X	X	X
300 and up	X	X	X	X	X	X	X	X	X	X	X	X	X

Men

Weight	5'4"	5'5"	5'6"	5'7"	5'8"	5'9"	5'10"	5'11"	6'0"	6'1"	6'2"	6'3"	6'4"	6'5"	6'6"	6'7" and up
up to 125	M	M	M	M	M	M	M	M	M	M	L	L	L	L	L	L
130	M	M	M	M	M	M	M	L	L	L	L	L	L	L	L	L
135	M	M	M	M	L	L	L	L	L	L	L	L	L	L	L	L
140	L	L	L	L	L	L	L	L	L	L	L	L	L	L	L	L
145	L	L	L	L	L	L	L	L	L	L	L	L	L	L	L	X
150	L	L	L	L	L	L	L	L	L	L	L	L	L	L	L	X
155	L	L	L	L	L	L	L	L	L	L	L	L	L	L	X	X
160	L	L	L	L	L	L	L	L	L	L	L	L	L	L	X	X
165	L	L	L	L	L	L	L	L	L	L	L	L	X	X	X	X
170	L	L	L	L	L	L	L	L	L	L	L	L	X	X	X	X
175	L	L	L	L	L	L	L	L	L	L	X	X	X	X	X	X
180	L	L	L	L	L	L	L	L	L	X	X	X	X	X	X	X
185	L	L	L	L	L	L	X	X	X	X	X	X	X	X	X	X
190	L	L	L	L	L	L	X	X	X	X	X	X	X	X	X	X
195	X	L	L	L	X	X	X	X	X	X	X	X	X	X	X	X
200	X	X	X	X	X	X	X	X	X	X	X	X	X	X	X	X
205	X	X	X	X	X	X	X	X	X	X	X	X	X	X	X	X
210	X	X	X	X	X	X	X	X	X	X	X	X	X	X	X	X
215	X	X	X	X	X	X	X	X	X	X	X	X	X	X	X	X
220	X	X	X	X	X	X	X	X	X	X	X	X	X	X	X	X
225	X	X	X	X	X	X	X	X	X	X	X	X	X	X	X	X
230	X	X	X	X	X	X	X	X	X	X	X	X	X	X	X	X
235	X	X	X	X	X	X	X	X	X	X	X	X	X	X	X	X
240	X	X	X	X	X	X	X	X	X	X	X	X	X	X	XX	XX
245	X	X	X	X	X	X	X	X	X	X	X	X	XX	XX	XX	XX
250	X	X	X	X	X	X	X	X	XX	XX	XX	XX	XX	XX	XX	XX
255	X	X	X	X	X	X	XX	XX	XX	XX	XX	XX	XX	XX	XX	XX
260	X	X	X	X	X	X	XX	XX	XX	XX	XX	XX	XX	XX	XX	XX
265	X	X	XX	XX	XX	XX	XX	XX	XX	XX	XX	XX	XX	XX	XX	XX
270	X	XX	XX	XX	XX	XX	XX	XX	XX	XX	XX	XX	XX	XX	XX	XX
275	X	XX	XX	XX	XX	XX	XX	XX	XX	XX	XX	XX	XX	XX	XX	XX
280	XX	XX	XX	XX	XX	XX	XX	XX	XX	XX	XX	XX	XX	XX	XX	XX
285	XX	XX	XX	XX	XX	XX	XX	XX	XX	XX	XX	XX	XX	XX	XX	XX
290	XX	XX	XX	XX	XX	XX	XX	XX	XX	XX	XX	XX	XX	XX	XX	XX
295	XX	XX	XX	XX	XX	XX	XX	XX	XX	XX	XX	XX	XX	XX	XX	XX
300	XX	XX	XX	XX	XX	XX	XX	XX	XX	XX	XX	XX	XX	XX	XX	XX
305	XX	XX	XX	XX	XX	XX	XX	XX	XX	XX	XX	XX	XX	XX	XX	XX

Height

310 and up

Protein and Carbohydrate Servings Lists

Protein Servings List
SMALL SERVING

Meats (includes beef, pork, lamb, poultry, and game)	3 ounces
Fish (includes saltwater, freshwater, and shellfish)	3 ounces
Eggs	3 whole eggs or 2 eggs + 2 whites
Cottage Cheese (or other curd-style cheeses)*	¾ cup
Tofu*	4 ounces
Eggs and Bacon, Ham, Sausage, or Fish	2 eggs + 1 ounce meat or fish or 2 strips bacon or 1 link sausage
To add hard cheeses*	Substitute 1 ounce cheese for 1 egg or 1 ounce meat or fish
Protein Powder*	about 20 grams per serving

Protein Servings List
MEDIUM SERVING

Meats (includes beef, pork, lamb, poultry, and game)	4 ounces
Fish (includes saltwater, freshwater, and shellfish)	4 ounces
Eggs	4 whole eggs or 2 eggs + 2 whites
Cottage Cheese (or other curd-style cheeses)*	1 cup

*These combination foods contain both protein *and* carbohydrate.

Tofu*	6 ounces
Eggs and Bacon, Ham, Sausage, or Fish	2 eggs + 2 whites + 1 ounce meat or fish or 2 strips bacon or 1 link sausage
To add hard cheeses*	Substitute 1 ounce cheese for 1 egg or 1 ounce meat or fish
Protein Powder*	about 27 grams per serving

Protein Servings List
LARGE SERVING

Meats (includes beef, pork, lamb, poultry, and game)	5 ounces
Fish (includes saltwater, freshwater, and shellfish)	5 ounces
Eggs	3 whole eggs + 4 whites
Cottage Cheese (or other curd-style cheeses)*	1¼ cups
Tofu*	7 ounces
Eggs and Bacon, Ham, Sausage, or Fish	4 eggs or 2 eggs + 2 whites and 1 ounce meat or fish or 2 strips bacon or 1 link sausage
To add hard cheeses*	Substitute 1 ounce cheese for 1 egg or 1 ounce meat or fish
Protein Powder*	about 34 grams per serving

Protein Servings List
EXTRA-LARGE SERVING

Meats (includes beef, pork, lamb, poultry, and game)	6 ounces
Fish (includes saltwater, freshwater, and shellfish)	6 ounces
Eggs	3 whole eggs + 6 whites
Cottage Cheese (or other curd-style cheeses)*	1½ cups
Tofu*	8 ounces

Eggs and Bacon, Ham, Sausage, or Fish	3 eggs + 3 ounces meat or fish or 4 strips bacon or 3 links sausage
To add hard cheeses*	Substitute 1 ounce cheese for 1 egg or for 1 ounce meat or fish
Protein Powder*	about 40 grams per serving

Protein Servings List
EXTRA-EXTRA-LARGE SERVING

Meats (includes beef, pork, lamb, poultry, and game)	8 ounces
Fish (includes saltwater, freshwater, and shellfish)	8 ounces
Eggs	4 whole eggs + 6 whites
Cottage Cheese (or other curd-style cheeses)*	2 cups
Tofu*	10 ounces
Eggs and Bacon, Ham, Sausage, or Fish	3 eggs + 4 ounces meat or fish or 6 strips bacon or 4 links sausage
To add hard cheeses*	Substitute 1 ounce cheese for 1 egg or for 1 ounce meat or fish
Protein Powder*	about 48 grams per serving

Carbohydrate Servings List
SMALL SERVING

During the corrective phase of your diet it's all-important to control your carb intake throughout the day. To construct your own meals at this earliest stage, you may choose two small carbohydrate servings at each meal or snack to stay within your carbohydrate limit. You might choose:

1 serving of fruit and 1 serving of vegetable—or—

1 serving of fruit and 1 serving of bread/cereal/grain—or—

1 serving of vegetable and 1 serving of bread/cereal/grain—or—

2 servings of fruit —or—

2 servings of vegetable

*These combination foods contain both protein *and* carbohydrate.

We would encourage you not to take both your servings as bread/cereal/grain as a general rule, since this category of foods is in most cases nutritionally pretty empty.

Assume all whole fruits and vegetables to be of medium size, unless specified otherwise.

Fruits

¼ apple
¼ cup applesauce
2 apricots
½ avocado
½ cup blackberries
⅓ cup blueberries
½ cup cantaloupe
5 whole sweet cherries
¼ cup sour cherries (canned)
⅓ cup cranberries (raw)
2 teaspoons jellied cranberry sauce
½ cup black currants
¼ cup canned fruit cocktail
¼ grapefruit
¼ cup canned grapefruit
⅓ cup grapes
½ guava
½ cup honeydew melon
½ kiwi
½ orange
1 passionfruit
½ peach
⅓ cup canned peaches (in water)
¼ pear
¼ cup pineapple (raw)
½ plum
1 prune
½ cup raspberries
¾ cup strawberries
½ cup strawberries (frozen, unsweetened)
½ tangerine
½ cup watermelon

Vegetables

¼ artichoke (whole)
¼ cup artichoke hearts
1–2 cups arugula
10 spears asparagus (fresh)
1 cup canned asparagus
1 cup bamboo shoots
½ cup black soybeans
½ cup beets
2 cups broccoli (raw)
1 cup broccoli (cooked)
1 cup broccoli/cauliflower (frozen)
5 brussels sprouts
1½ cups cabbage (raw)
1 cup cabbage (cooked)
1 medium carrot (raw)
½ cup carrots (cooked)
2 cups cauliflower (raw)
1½ cups cauliflower (cooked)
4 stalks celery (raw)
¾ cup celery (cooked)

Vegetables (continued)

¾ cup chard (cooked)

(unlimited) chives

⅓ cup homemade coleslaw

½ cucumber (raw)

¾ cup eggplant (cooked)

1–2 cups endive (raw)

¾ cup fennel (fresh)

3 cloves garlic

¼ cup sliced ginger (raw)

1 cup green beans (cooked)

1 cup green (spring) onions (raw)

½ cup greens (cooked)

½ cup kale (cooked)

¼ cup kelp (raw)

½ cup leeks (cooked)

(unlimited) lettuce

2 cups mushrooms (raw)

¾ cup mushrooms (cooked)

½ cup okra

½ cup onions (raw)

¼ cup onions (cooked)

(unlimited) parsley

⅓ cup green peas

½ cup chile peppers (canned)

1 whole chile pepper (raw)

½ sweet (bell) pepper (large, raw)

½ cup sweet (bell) pepper (cooked)

(unlimited) radicchio

(unlimited) radishes

½ cup rhubarb (cooked)

⅓ cup rutabaga (cooked)

½ cup sauerkraut

3 tablespoons shallots (raw)

(unlimited) spinach

½ cup spaghetti squash (cooked)

½ cup summer squash (cooked)
  (crookneck, scallop, zucchini)

⅓ cup winter squash (cooked)
  (acorn, butternut, hubbard)

2 tomatillos (raw)

1 tomato (raw)

½ cup tomato (canned)

1 cup turnips (boiled)

¼ cup water chestnuts (canned)

5 whole water chestnuts (canned)

½ cup wax beans

Bread, Cereal, and Grains

1 slice bread (commercial
  low-carb)

2–4 saltine crackers
  (commercial fat-free)[1]

10 oyster crackers

1 Triscuit

2 Wasa crisp bread

2 Melba toast

8 Cheese Nips

½ rice cake

⅛ cup rice

1 La Tortilla Factory low-carb
  tortilla[2]

---

1. Be aware that virtually all commercially baked goods contain transfats, which have been shown to be a health hazard. Where possible, buy fat-free baked goods to avoid these bad fats, or make your own baked goods using the recipes in *The Low-Carb Comfort Food Cookbook*.
2. Available in many stores.

Carbohydrate Servings List
MODERATE SERVING

As you approach your goal weight and/or target values for blood pressure, blood sugar, and blood lipids, you can begin to increase the amount of carbohydrate you're eating. As a guideline for constructing your own slightly higher-carb meals, you may choose two medium carbohydrate servings at each meal or snack. If you see your weight begin to sneak up again, drop back to the small level for a bit longer. A meal in the medium-carb range might include:

1 serving of fruit and 1 serving of vegetable—or—

1 serving of fruit and 1 serving of bread/cereal/grain—or—

1 serving of vegetable and 1 serving of bread/cereal/grain—or—

2 servings of fruit—or—

2 servings of vegetable

We would not encourage you to take both your servings as bread/cereal/grain as a general rule, since this category of foods is in most cases nutritionally pretty empty.

Assume all whole fruits or vegetables to be of medium size, unless specified otherwise.

Fruits

½ apple
½ cup applesauce
3 apricots (raw)
8 apricot halves (canned)
1 avocado
½ banana (small)
¾ cup blackberries
½ cup blueberries
¾ cup cantaloupe
10 whole sweet cherries
½ cup sour cherries (canned)
¾ cup cranberries (raw)

1 tbsp. jellied cranberry sauce
¾ cup black currants
1 date (whole)
1 fig
½ cup fruit cocktail (in water)
½ grapefruit (fresh)
⅓ cup canned grapefruit
½ cup grapes
1 guava
½ cup honeydew melon
1 kiwi
⅓ cup mandarin orange (in water)

Fruits (continued)

¼ cup mango

½ nectarine

¾ orange

¼ papaya

2 passionfruit

1 peach

½ cup canned peaches (in water)

1 peach half (dried)

½ pear

½ pear, Asian

¼ cup pineapple

1 persimmon

1 plum

¼ pomegranate

2 prunes

½ quince

1 cup raspberries

1 cup strawberries (fresh)

¾ cup strawberries (frozen, unsweetened)

1 tangerine (medium)

¾ cup watermelon

Vegetables

1 cup alfalfa sprouts

½ artichoke (whole)

½ cup artichoke hearts

(unlimited) arugula

20 spears asparagus (fresh)

1½ cups canned asparagus

2 cups bamboo shoots

⅓ cup beans, dried (cooked)

¾ cup beets (boiled)

¼ cup beets, pickled (canned)

1 cup black soybeans

⅓ cup black eyed peas or cow-peas (canned)

4 cups broccoli (raw)

2 cups broccoli (cooked)

1½ cups broccoli and carrots (frozen)

2 cups broccoli and cauliflower (frozen)

10 brussels sprouts (fresh)

⅓ cup butter beans (canned)

3 cups cabbage (raw)

2 cups cabbage (cooked)

2 carrots (raw)

¾ cup carrots (cooked)

4 cups cauliflower (raw)

2 cups cauliflower (cooked)

(unlimited) stalks celery (raw)

1½ cups celery (cooked)

1 cup chard (cooked)

¼ cup chickpeas or garbanzo beans (cooked)

(unlimited) chives

½ cup homemade coleslaw

¼ cup corn (cooked)

1 cucumber (raw)

1 cup eggplant (cooked)

4 cups endive (raw)

1 cup fennel (fresh)

(unlimited) cloves garlic

½ cup sliced ginger (raw)

1½ cups green beans (cooked)

2 cups green (spring) onions (raw)

1½ cups greens (beet, collard, turnip, mustard) (cooked)

1 cup kale (cooked)

½ cup kelp (raw)

1 cup leeks (cooked)

(unlimited) lettuce

(unlimited) mushrooms (raw)

2 cups mushrooms (cooked)

¾ cup okra

¾ cup onions (raw)

½ cup onions (cooked)

(unlimited) parsley

½ cup green peas

1 cup chile peppers (canned)

2 whole chile peppers (raw)

1 sweet (bell) pepper (small, raw)

1½ cups sweet (bell) pepper (cooked)

(unlimited) radicchio

(unlimited) radishes

1 cup rhubarb (cooked)

½ cup rutabaga (cooked)

¾ cup sauerkraut

⅓ cup shallots (raw)

(unlimited) spinach

1 cup spaghetti squash (cooked)

1 cup summer squash (cooked) (crookneck, scallop, zucchini)

⅔ cup winter squash (cooked) (acorn, butternut, hubbard)

5 tomatillos (medium, raw)

2 tomatoes (medium, raw)

1 cup tomato (canned)

¼ cup sundried tomato

1 cup turnips (cooked)

½ cup water chestnuts (canned) or 10 whole water chestnuts (canned)

1 cup wax beans

¼ cup yams (cooked)

Bread, Cereal, and Grains

1 small biscuit or roll (¾ ounce)

1½ slices bread (commercial low-carb)

4 saltine crackers (commercial fat-free)

20 oyster crackers (commercial fat-free)

½ hamburger or hot dog bun (commercial fat-free)

3 Triscuits

5 Wasa crisp bread

4 Melba toast

15 Cheese Nips

½ small pita pocket

1 rice cake

¼ cup rice

2 La Tortilla Factory low-carb tortillas[3]

1 taco shell (commercial)

3. Available in many stores.

Carbohydrate Servings List
LARGE SERVING

During the maintenance phase of your diet, you may pretty freely choose to eat from any of the serving lists in whatever combination suits you. Remember that the total carbohydrate content of a meal or snack will be the sum of all the fruit, vegetables, breads, cereals, grains, nuts, and dairy products it contains. For a simple guide to constructing your own meals, begin by choosing two large carbohydrate servings at each meal or snack and see how you do, increasing your carb intake from these good foods as you feel comfortable. Remember that if your weight begins to climb or your blood pressure, blood sugar, or blood lipids begin to rise, you must cut back again on the amount of carbohydrate that you're eating. Drop back to the strict definition of a large serving first. If necessary, go back to the medium or even to the small level for a few days and recover your weight, pressure, or return blood test values to normal before advancing again.

As you enter maintenance, begin by eating two large servings of carb at each meal or snack. This could include:

1 serving of fruit and 1 serving of vegetable—or—

1 serving of fruit and 1 serving of bread/cereal/grain—or—

1 serving of vegetable and 1 serving of bread/cereal/grain—or—

2 servings of fruit—or—

2 servings of vegetable

We would not encourage you to take both your servings as bread/cereal/grain as a general rule, since this category of foods is in most cases nutritionally pretty empty.

Assume all whole fruits or vegetables to be of medium size, unless specified otherwise.

Fruits

¾ apple	2 avocado
¾ cup applesauce	½ banana (medium)
4 apricots (raw)	1¼ cups blackberries
12 apricot halves (canned)	¾ cup blueberries

1 cup cantaloupe

15 whole sweet cherries

¾ cup sour cherries (canned)

1 cup cranberries (raw)

2 tbsp. jellied cranberry sauce

1 cup black currants

2 dates (whole)

1½ figs

¾ cup fruit cocktail (in water)

¾ grapefruit (fresh)

⅔ cup canned grapefruit

1 cup grapes

1½ guavas

1 cup honeydew melon

1½ kiwis

½ cup mandarin orange (in water)

½ cup mango

1 nectarine

1 orange

½ papaya

3 passionfruits

1½ peaches

1 cup canned peaches (in water)

1½ peach halves (dried)

¾ pear

1 pear, Asian

¾ cup pineapple

1½ persimmons

1½ plums

½ pomegranate

3 prunes

1 quince

1¾ cups raspberries

2 cups strawberries (fresh)

1½ cups strawberries (frozen, unsweetened)

1½ tangerines (medium)

1 cup watermelon

Vegetables

(unlimited) alfalfa sprouts

1 artichoke (whole)

¾ cup artichoke hearts

(unlimited) arugula

25 spears asparagus (fresh)

2 cups canned asparagus

3 cups bamboo shoots

½ cup beans, dried (cooked)

1 cup beets (boiled)

⅓ cup beets, pickled (canned)

1½ cups black soybeans

½ cup black eyed peas or cow-peas (canned)

(unlimited) broccoli (raw)

3 cups broccoli (cooked)

2 cups broccoli and carrots (frozen)

2½ cups broccoli and cauliflower (frozen)

15 brussels sprouts (fresh)

½ cup butter beans (canned)

(unlimited) cabbage (raw)

3 cups cabbage (cooked)

3 carrots (raw)

1 cup carrots (cooked)

5 cups cauliflower (raw)

3 cups cauliflower (cooked)

Vegetables (continued)

(unlimited) stalks celery (raw)

2 cups celery (cooked)

1 cup chard (cooked)

⅓ cup chickpeas or garbanzo beans (cooked)

(unlimited) chives

1 cup homemade coleslaw

⅓ cup corn (cooked)

2 cucumbers (raw)

2 cups eggplant (cooked)

(unlimited) endive (raw)

2 cups fennel (fresh)

(unlimited) cloves garlic

¾ cup sliced ginger (raw)

2 cups green beans (cooked)

(unlimited) green (spring) onions (raw)

2 cups greens (beet, collard, turnip, mustard) (cooked)

2 cups kale (cooked)

⅔ cup kelp (raw)

1½ cups leeks (cooked)

(unlimited) lettuce

(unlimited) mushrooms (raw)

3 cups mushrooms (cooked)

1 cup okra

¾ cup onions (raw)

½ cup onions (cooked)

(unlimited) parsley

¾ cup green peas

1¾ cups chile peppers (canned)

3 whole chile peppers (raw)

1 sweet (bell) pepper (large, raw)

2 cups sweet (bell) pepper (cooked)

¼ potato, baked with skin

⅓ cup potato, mashed

½ cup pumpkin

(unlimited) radicchio

(unlimited) radishes

1½ cups rhubarb (cooked)

1 cup rutabaga (cooked)

1 cup sauerkraut

(unlimited) shallots (raw)

(unlimited) spinach

1½ cups spaghetti squash (cooked)

3 cups summer squash (cooked) (crookneck, scallop, zucchini)

1 cup winter squash (cooked) (acorn, butternut, hubbard)

7 tomatillos (medium, raw)

3 tomatoes (medium, raw)

1½ cups tomato (canned)

½ cup sundried tomato

3 cups turnips (cooked)

¾ cup water chestnuts (canned)

15 whole water chestnuts (canned)

1½ cups wax beans

⅓ cup yams (cooked)

Bread/Cereal/Grain

½ bagel (medium)

1 medium biscuit or roll
(1 ounce)

2 slices bread (commercial
low-carb)

6 saltine crackers (commercial
fat-free)[4]

25 oyster crackers (commercial
fat-free)

⅓ cup couscous (cooked)

½ English muffin (commercial
fat-free)

1 hamburger or hot dog bun
(commercial fat-free)

5 Triscuits

7 Wasa crisp bread

6 Melba toast

25 Cheese Nips

1 small pita pocket

2 rice cakes

⅓ cup rice

3 La Tortilla Factory low-carb
tortillas[5]

1 fajita wrap (small,
commercial)

2 taco shells (commercial)

1 waffle (small, frozen,
commercial)

---

4. Be aware that virtually all commercially baked goods contain transfats, which have been shown to be a health hazard. Where possible, buy fat-free baked goods to avoid these bad fats, or make your own baked goods using the recipes in *The Low-Carb Comfort Food Cookbook*.
5. Available in many stores.

Meal Planner Worksheet

(photocopy as needed)

Protein Serving Size   _____ (S, M, L, XL, XXL)

Carbohydrate Serving Size _____ (small, moderate, large)

	Yes	No
Did you take your multivitamin/mineral?	☐	☐
Did you take extra potassium/magnesium?	☐	☐

	What you planned to eat	What you actually ate
Breakfast:		
Protein serving	_____	_____
	_____	_____
Carb serving	_____	_____
	_____	_____
Fluid (ounces)	_____	_____
Lunch:		
Protein serving	_____	_____
	_____	_____
Carb serving	_____	_____
	_____	_____
Fluid (ounces)	_____	_____
Snack:		
	_____	_____
	_____	_____
	_____	_____
	_____	_____
Dinner:		
Protein serving	_____	_____
	_____	_____
Carb serving	_____	_____
	_____	_____
Fluid (ounces)	_____	_____

The Staying Power LifePlanner

Welcome to a new way of living and eating! One of the best tools for making your plan work for you is to put it in writing. We've designed the LifePlanner with this goal in mind. By diligently using it to record everything you put into your mouth—every bite, every sip, all vitamin and mineral supplements, even medications—you will substantially enhance your odds of successfully rehabilitating your health and fitness. Studies have shown that simply keeping a faithful record of your activities increases the likelihood of success in dieting or any important behavioral change. Be brutally honest in keeping your records—after all, they're there to help you, not indict you.

For each day of the year you'll find a space to record your meals and optional snacks, as well as your exercise (both aerobic and resistance) and intake of fluids and supplements. There's a place to total each meal's carbohydrate intake and a space for the day's carb total.

We've divided the Staying Power LifePlanner into week-long intervals, beginning with January 1 to January 7. Depending on the year, those particular days may not constitute a Monday through Sunday week, because we designed your LifePlanner to be universal from year to year. No matter when you begin your Staying Power LifePlanner regimen, simply turn to the day of the year in question and circle the day of the week. That date might not be the start of a seven-day journal interval, but that's okay. Just begin on the correct date, finish the remaining days that week, and by the following week, you'll be in sync with the planner. You'll fill the remainder of that first week's entries at the end of your Staying Power year.

In the back of your LifePlanner, we've included a section for you to record and track your blood pressure and laboratory values throughout the year, so you can easily see your progress. And each weekly interval brings you a new motivating and inspiring quote and a Staying Power tip.

We hope that using the Staying Power LifePlanner will make sticking to your commitment easier.

Best of luck in reclaiming your health and fitness.

JANUARY 1	BREAKFAST	LUNCH	DINNER	SNACKS
S M T W T F S Carbohydrate Total per Meal: B _____ L _____ D _____ S _____				
Daily Carbohydrate	Fluids: oz.	Fluids: oz.	Fluids: oz.	Fluids: oz.
Total: _____	Vit / Min / Supp:			

JANUARY 2	BREAKFAST	LUNCH	DINNER	SNACKS
S M T W T F S Carbohydrate Total per Meal: B _____ L _____ D _____ S _____				
Daily Carbohydrate	Fluids: oz.	Fluids: oz.	Fluids: oz.	Fluids: oz.
Total: _____	Vit / Min / Supp:			

JANUARY 3	BREAKFAST	LUNCH	DINNER	SNACKS
S M T W T F S Carbohydrate Total per Meal: B _____ L _____ D _____ S _____				
Daily Carbohydrate	Fluids: oz.	Fluids: oz.	Fluids: oz.	Fluids: oz.
Total: _____	Vit / Min / Supp:			

JANUARY 4	BREAKFAST	LUNCH	DINNER	SNACKS
S M T W T F S Carbohydrate Total per Meal: B _____ L _____ D _____ S _____				
Daily Carbohydrate	Fluids: oz.	Fluids: oz.	Fluids: oz.	Fluids: oz.
Total: _____	Vit / Min / Supp:			

EXERCISE GOALS: _____

EXERCISE DONE: _____

JANUARY 5	BREAKFAST	LUNCH	DINNER	SNACKS
S M T W T F S Carbohydrate Total per Meal: B _____ L _____ D _____ S _____				
Daily Carbohydrate Total: _____	Fluids: oz.	Fluids: oz.	Fluids: oz.	Fluids: oz.
	Vit / Min / Supp:			

JANUARY 6	BREAKFAST	LUNCH	DINNER	SNACKS
S M T W T F S Carbohydrate Total per Meal: B _____ L _____ D _____ S _____				
Daily Carbohydrate Total: _____	Fluids: oz.	Fluids: oz.	Fluids: oz.	Fluids: oz.
	Vit / Min / Supp:			

JANUARY 7	BREAKFAST	LUNCH	DINNER	SNACKS
S M T W T F S Carbohydrate Total per Meal: B _____ L _____ D _____ S _____				
Daily Carbohydrate Total: _____	Fluids: oz.	Fluids: oz.	Fluids: oz.	Fluids: oz.
	Vit / Min / Supp:			

TIP   As an aperitif, fifteen to twenty minutes before a meal drink 6 to 8 oz. of sparkling water with a lime slice. When finished with your meal, drink a cup of hot herb tea or green tea. It is good for you and adds to your feeling of satisfaction.

QUOTE   "On any journey, we must find out where we are before we can plan the first step." — *Kathy Boevink*

GOAL FOR THE WEEK:

STATISTICS	weight	waist"	hips"
Beginning:	_____	_____	_____
End:	_____	_____	_____

JANUARY 8	BREAKFAST	LUNCH	DINNER	SNACKS
S M T W T F S Carbohydrate Total per Meal: B _____ L _____ D _____ S _____				
Daily Carbohydrate Total: _____	Fluids: _____ oz.	Fluids: _____ oz.	Fluids: _____ oz.	Fluids: _____ oz.
	Vit / Min / Supp:			

JANUARY 9	BREAKFAST	LUNCH	DINNER	SNACKS
S M T W T F S Carbohydrate Total per Meal: B _____ L _____ D _____ S _____				
Daily Carbohydrate Total: _____	Fluids: _____ oz.	Fluids: _____ oz.	Fluids: _____ oz.	Fluids: _____ oz.
	Vit / Min / Supp:			

JANUARY 10	BREAKFAST	LUNCH	DINNER	SNACKS
S M T W T F S Carbohydrate Total per Meal: B _____ L _____ D _____ S _____				
Daily Carbohydrate Total: _____	Fluids: _____ oz.	Fluids: _____ oz.	Fluids: _____ oz.	Fluids: _____ oz.
	Vit / Min / Supp:			

JANUARY 11	BREAKFAST	LUNCH	DINNER	SNACKS
S M T W T F S Carbohydrate Total per Meal: B _____ L _____ D _____ S _____				
Daily Carbohydrate Total: _____	Fluids: _____ oz.	Fluids: _____ oz.	Fluids: _____ oz.	Fluids: _____ oz.
	Vit / Min / Supp:			

EXERCISE GOALS: _____

EXERCISE DONE: _____

148

JANUARY 12	BREAKFAST	LUNCH	DINNER	SNACKS
S M T W T F S Carbohydrate Total per Meal: B _____ L _____ D _____ S _____				
Daily Carbohydrate Total: _____	Fluids: ___ oz.	Fluids: ___ oz.	Fluids: ___ oz.	Fluids: ___ oz.
	Vit / Min / Supp:			

JANUARY 13	BREAKFAST	LUNCH	DINNER	SNACKS
S M T W T F S Carbohydrate Total per Meal: B _____ L _____ D _____ S _____				
Daily Carbohydrate Total: _____	Fluids: ___ oz.	Fluids: ___ oz.	Fluids: ___ oz.	Fluids: ___ oz.
	Vit / Min / Supp:			

JANUARY 14	BREAKFAST	LUNCH	DINNER	SNACKS
S M T W T F S Carbohydrate Total per Meal: B _____ L _____ D _____ S _____				
Daily Carbohydrate Total: _____	Fluids: ___ oz.	Fluids: ___ oz.	Fluids: ___ oz.	Fluids: ___ oz.
	Vit / Min / Supp:			

TIP Create a soothing bath for yourself after exercise by making a sachet using 1 washcloth, ½ cup Epsom salts, and ½ sliced lemon. Spread out the washcloth and add the Epsom salts and lemon slices. Tie the mixture up by tying a knot in the opposing corners of the washcloth. Drop your sachet in a tub of hot water and enjoy.

QUOTE "Make everything as simple as possible, but not simpler." — *Albert Einstein*

GOAL FOR THE WEEK:

STATISTICS	weight	waist"	hips"
Beginning:	_____	_____	_____
End:	_____	_____	_____

JANUARY 15	BREAKFAST	LUNCH	DINNER	SNACKS
S M T W T F S Carbohydrate Total per Meal: B _____ L _____ D _____ S _____ Daily Carbohydrate Total: _____				
	Fluids: oz.	Fluids: oz.	Fluids: oz.	Fluids: oz.
	Vit / Min / Supp:			

JANUARY 16	BREAKFAST	LUNCH	DINNER	SNACKS
S M T W T F S Carbohydrate Total per Meal: B _____ L _____ D _____ S _____ Daily Carbohydrate Total: _____				
	Fluids: oz.	Fluids: oz.	Fluids: oz.	Fluids: oz.
	Vit / Min / Supp:			

JANUARY 17	BREAKFAST	LUNCH	DINNER	SNACKS
S M T W T F S Carbohydrate Total per Meal: B _____ L _____ D _____ S _____ Daily Carbohydrate Total: _____				
	Fluids: oz.	Fluids: oz.	Fluids: oz.	Fluids: oz.
	Vit / Min / Supp:			

JANUARY 18	BREAKFAST	LUNCH	DINNER	SNACKS
S M T W T F S Carbohydrate Total per Meal: B _____ L _____ D _____ S _____ Daily Carbohydrate Total: _____				
	Fluids: oz.	Fluids: oz.	Fluids: oz.	Fluids: oz.
	Vit / Min / Supp:			

EXERCISE GOALS: _____

EXERCISE DONE: _____

JANUARY 19	BREAKFAST	LUNCH	DINNER	SNACKS
S M T W T F S Carbohydrate Total per Meal: B _____ L _____ D _____ S _____ Daily Carbohydrate Total: _____				
	Fluids: _____ oz.	Fluids: _____ oz.	Fluids: _____ oz.	Fluids: _____ oz.
	Vit / Min / Supp:			

JANUARY 20	BREAKFAST	LUNCH	DINNER	SNACKS
S M T W T F S Carbohydrate Total per Meal: B _____ L _____ D _____ S _____ Daily Carbohydrate Total: _____				
	Fluids: _____ oz.	Fluids: _____ oz.	Fluids: _____ oz.	Fluids: _____ oz.
	Vit / Min / Supp:			

JANUARY 21	BREAKFAST	LUNCH	DINNER	SNACKS
S M T W T F S Carbohydrate Total per Meal: B _____ L _____ D _____ S _____ Daily Carbohydrate Total: _____				
	Fluids: _____ oz.	Fluids: _____ oz.	Fluids: _____ oz.	Fluids: _____ oz.
	Vit / Min / Supp:			

TIP   Pork rinds are a crunchy, satisfying snack. To create a fine spreading sauce for them, roast several cloves of garlic and puree. Cut the top portion off a bulb of garlic, drizzle a small amount of olive oil over the top, seal in a pouch of foil, and bake in a 325-degree oven for 20 minutes. Remove from the oven, squeeze all the roasted garlic from the cloves, add a small amount of olive oil, mix, and spread on the pork rinds.

QUOTE   "Limited expectations yield only limited results." — *Susan Laurson Willig*

GOAL FOR THE WEEK:

STATISTICS	weight	waist"	hips"
Beginning:	_____	_____	_____
End:	_____	_____	_____

JANUARY 22	BREAKFAST	LUNCH	DINNER	SNACKS
S M T W T F S Carbohydrate Total per Meal: B _____ L _____ D _____ S _____				
Daily Carbohydrate Total: _____	Fluids: oz.	Fluids: oz.	Fluids: oz.	Fluids: oz.
	Vit / Min / Supp:			

JANUARY 23	BREAKFAST	LUNCH	DINNER	SNACKS
S M T W T F S Carbohydrate Total per Meal: B _____ L _____ D _____ S _____				
Daily Carbohydrate Total: _____	Fluids: oz.	Fluids: oz.	Fluids: oz.	Fluids: oz.
	Vit / Min / Supp:			

JANUARY 24	BREAKFAST	LUNCH	DINNER	SNACKS
S M T W T F S Carbohydrate Total per Meal: B _____ L _____ D _____ S _____				
Daily Carbohydrate Total: _____	Fluids: oz.	Fluids: oz.	Fluids: oz.	Fluids: oz.
	Vit / Min / Supp:			

JANUARY 25	BREAKFAST	LUNCH	DINNER	SNACKS
S M T W T F S Carbohydrate Total per Meal: B _____ L _____ D _____ S _____				
Daily Carbohydrate Total: _____	Fluids: oz.	Fluids: oz.	Fluids: oz.	Fluids: oz.
	Vit / Min / Supp:			

EXERCISE GOALS: _____

EXERCISE DONE: _____

JANUARY 26	BREAKFAST	LUNCH	DINNER	SNACKS
S M T W T F S Carbohydrate Total per Meal: B _____ L _____ D _____ S _____				
Daily Carbohydrate Total: _____	Fluids: oz. Vit / Min / Supp:	Fluids: oz.	Fluids: oz.	Fluids: oz.

JANUARY 27	BREAKFAST	LUNCH	DINNER	SNACKS
S M T W T F S Carbohydrate Total per Meal: B _____ L _____ D _____ S _____				
Daily Carbohydrate Total: _____	Fluids: oz. Vit / Min / Supp:	Fluids: oz.	Fluids: oz.	Fluids: oz.

JANUARY 28	BREAKFAST	LUNCH	DINNER	SNACKS
S M T W T F S Carbohydrate Total per Meal: B _____ L _____ D _____ S _____				
Daily Carbohydrate Total: _____	Fluids: oz. Vit / Min / Supp:	Fluids: oz.	Fluids: oz.	Fluids: oz.

TIP   Remember, it's your carbohydrate intake that drives your blood insulin levels and your ability (or inability) to burn fat.

QUOTE   "Most of the shadows of this life are caused by standing in one's own sunshine." — *Ralph Waldo Emerson*

GOAL FOR THE WEEK:

STATISTICS   weight   waist"   hips"
Beginning: _____   _____   _____
End: _____   _____   _____

JANUARY 29	BREAKFAST	LUNCH	DINNER	SNACKS
S M T W T F S Carbohydrate Total per Meal: B _____ L _____ D _____ S _____ Daily Carbohydrate Total: _____				
	Fluids: oz.	Fluids: oz.	Fluids: oz.	Fluids: oz.
	Vit / Min / Supp:			

JANUARY 30	BREAKFAST	LUNCH	DINNER	SNACKS
S M T W T F S Carbohydrate Total per Meal: B _____ L _____ D _____ S _____ Daily Carbohydrate Total: _____				
	Fluids: oz.	Fluids: oz.	Fluids: oz.	Fluids: oz.
	Vit / Min / Supp:			

JANUARY 31	BREAKFAST	LUNCH	DINNER	SNACKS
S M T W T F S Carbohydrate Total per Meal: B _____ L _____ D _____ S _____ Daily Carbohydrate Total: _____				
	Fluids: oz.	Fluids: oz.	Fluids: oz.	Fluids: oz.
	Vit / Min / Supp:			

FEBRUARY 1	BREAKFAST	LUNCH	DINNER	SNACKS
S M T W T F S Carbohydrate Total per Meal: B _____ L _____ D _____ S _____ Daily Carbohydrate Total: _____				
	Fluids: oz.	Fluids: oz.	Fluids: oz.	Fluids: oz.
	Vit / Min / Supp:			

EXERCISE GOALS: _____

EXERCISE DONE: _____

154

FEBRUARY 2	BREAKFAST	LUNCH	DINNER	SNACKS
S M T W T F S Carbohydrate Total per Meal: B _____ L _____ D _____ S _____				
Daily Carbohydrate Total: _____	Fluids: _____ oz.	Fluids: _____ oz.	Fluids: _____ oz.	Fluids: _____ oz.
	Vit / Min / Supp:			

FEBRUARY 3	BREAKFAST	LUNCH	DINNER	SNACKS
S M T W T F S Carbohydrate Total per Meal: B _____ L _____ D _____ S _____				
Daily Carbohydrate Total: _____	Fluids: _____ oz.	Fluids: _____ oz.	Fluids: _____ oz.	Fluids: _____ oz.
	Vit / Min / Supp:			

FEBRUARY 4	BREAKFAST	LUNCH	DINNER	SNACKS
S M T W T F S Carbohydrate Total per Meal: B _____ L _____ D _____ S _____				
Daily Carbohydrate Total: _____	Fluids: _____ oz.	Fluids: _____ oz.	Fluids: _____ oz.	Fluids: _____ oz.
	Vit / Min / Supp:			

TIP   If you find you have strayed from your maintenance diet, don't throw in the towel! Just return to the corrective phase for three days or until you are back to the weight you were before you fell off the wagon. Then move to transition for four days. Then move on to maintenance.

QUOTE   "Only those who dare, truly live." — *Ruth P. Freedman*

GOAL FOR THE WEEK:

STATISTICS	weight	waist"	hips"
Beginning:	_____	_____	_____
End:	_____	_____	_____

FEBRUARY 5	BREAKFAST	LUNCH	DINNER	SNACKS
S M T W T F S Carbohydrate Total per Meal: B _____ L _____ D _____ S _____				
Daily Carbohydrate Total: _____	Fluids: oz.	Fluids: oz.	Fluids: oz.	Fluids: oz.
	Vit/Min/Supp:			

FEBRUARY 6	BREAKFAST	LUNCH	DINNER	SNACKS
S M T W T F S Carbohydrate Total per Meal: B _____ L _____ D _____ S _____				
Daily Carbohydrate Total: _____	Fluids: oz.	Fluids: oz.	Fluids: oz.	Fluids: oz.
	Vit/Min/Supp:			

FEBRUARY 7	BREAKFAST	LUNCH	DINNER	SNACKS
S M T W T F S Carbohydrate Total per Meal: B _____ L _____ D _____ S _____				
Daily Carbohydrate Total: _____	Fluids: oz.	Fluids: oz.	Fluids: oz.	Fluids: oz.
	Vit/Min/Supp:			

FEBRUARY 8	BREAKFAST	LUNCH	DINNER	SNACKS
S M T W T F S Carbohydrate Total per Meal: B _____ L _____ D _____ S _____				
Daily Carbohydrate Total: _____	Fluids: oz.	Fluids: oz.	Fluids: oz.	Fluids: oz.
	Vit/Min/Supp:			

EXERCISE GOALS: _____

EXERCISE DONE: _____

FEBRUARY 9	BREAKFAST	LUNCH	DINNER	SNACKS
S M T W T F S Carbohydrate Total per Meal: B _____ L _____ D _____ S _____				
Daily Carbohydrate Total: _____	Fluids: ____ oz.	Fluids: ____ oz.	Fluids: ____ oz.	Fluids: ____ oz.
	Vit / Min / Supp:			

FEBRUARY 10	BREAKFAST	LUNCH	DINNER	SNACKS
S M T W T F S Carbohydrate Total per Meal: B _____ L _____ D _____ S _____				
Daily Carbohydrate Total: _____	Fluids: ____ oz.	Fluids: ____ oz.	Fluids: ____ oz.	Fluids: ____ oz.
	Vit / Min / Supp:			

FEBRUARY 11	BREAKFAST	LUNCH	DINNER	SNACKS
S M T W T F S Carbohydrate Total per Meal: B _____ L _____ D _____ S _____				
Daily Carbohydrate Total: _____	Fluids: ____ oz.	Fluids: ____ oz.	Fluids: ____ oz.	Fluids: ____ oz.
	Vit / Min / Supp:			

TIP   Eating 25 grams of fiber each day is important. As you look at your carbohydrate chart, you should note that the foods with the most fiber are usually the ones that have the biggest portions with the least carb grams.

QUOTE   "Courage is the price that life extracts for granting peace." — *Amelia Earhart*

GOAL FOR THE WEEK:

STATISTICS	weight	waist"	hips"
Beginning:	_____	_____	_____
End:	_____	_____	_____

157

FEBRUARY 12	BREAKFAST	LUNCH	DINNER	SNACKS
S M T W T F S Carbohydrate Total per Meal: B _____ L _____ D _____ S _____				
Daily Carbohydrate Total: _____	Fluids: ____ oz.	Fluids: ____ oz.	Fluids: ____ oz.	Fluids: ____ oz.
	Vit / Min / Supp:			

FEBRUARY 13	BREAKFAST	LUNCH	DINNER	SNACKS
S M T W T F S Carbohydrate Total per Meal: B _____ L _____ D _____ S _____				
Daily Carbohydrate Total: _____	Fluids: ____ oz.	Fluids: ____ oz.	Fluids: ____ oz.	Fluids: ____ oz.
	Vit / Min / Supp:			

FEBRUARY 14	BREAKFAST	LUNCH	DINNER	SNACKS
S M T W T F S Carbohydrate Total per Meal: B _____ L _____ D _____ S _____				
Daily Carbohydrate Total: _____	Fluids: ____ oz.	Fluids: ____ oz.	Fluids: ____ oz.	Fluids: ____ oz.
	Vit / Min / Supp:			

FEBRUARY 15	BREAKFAST	LUNCH	DINNER	SNACKS
S M T W T F S Carbohydrate Total per Meal: B _____ L _____ D _____ S _____				
Daily Carbohydrate Total: _____	Fluids: ____ oz.	Fluids: ____ oz.	Fluids: ____ oz.	Fluids: ____ oz.
	Vit / Min / Supp:			

EXERCISE GOALS: _____

EXERCISE DONE: _____

FEBRUARY 16	BREAKFAST	LUNCH	DINNER	SNACKS
S M T W T F S Carbohydrate Total per Meal: B _____ L _____ D _____ S _____				
Daily Carbohydrate Total: _____	Fluids: _____ oz. Vit / Min / Supp:	Fluids: _____ oz.	Fluids: _____ oz.	Fluids: _____ oz.

FEBRUARY 17	BREAKFAST	LUNCH	DINNER	SNACKS
S M T W T F S Carbohydrate Total per Meal: B _____ L _____ D _____ S _____				
Daily Carbohydrate Total: _____	Fluids: _____ oz. Vit / Min / Supp:	Fluids: _____ oz.	Fluids: _____ oz.	Fluids: _____ oz.

FEBRUARY 18	BREAKFAST	LUNCH	DINNER	SNACKS
S M T W T F S Carbohydrate Total per Meal: B _____ L _____ D _____ S _____				
Daily Carbohydrate Total: _____	Fluids: _____ oz. Vit / Min / Supp:	Fluids: _____ oz.	Fluids: _____ oz.	Fluids: _____ oz.

TIP   Wine, alcohol, and beer are permissible as long as you count the carbs! Dry white (3 oz.) or red wine (3 oz.) and light beer (12 oz.) will cost you 3 or 4 grams, but are still reasonable choices as long as you count them in your daily totals. Hard liquor can have a more pronounced effect on your insulin levels. Wine—in moderation—can help improve insulin sensitivity.

QUOTE   "There's a period of life where we swallow a knowledge of ourselves and it becomes either good or sour inside." — *Pearl Bailey*

GOAL FOR THE WEEK:

STATISTICS	weight	waist"	hips"
Beginning:	_____	_____	_____
End:	_____	_____	_____

FEBRUARY 19	BREAKFAST	LUNCH	DINNER	SNACKS
S M T W T F S Carbohydrate Total per Meal: B _____ L _____ D _____ S _____ Daily Carbohydrate Total: _____				
	Fluids: oz.	Fluids: oz.	Fluids: oz.	Fluids: oz.
	Vit / Min / Supp:			

FEBRUARY 20	BREAKFAST	LUNCH	DINNER	SNACKS
S M T W T F S Carbohydrate Total per Meal: B _____ L _____ D _____ S _____ Daily Carbohydrate Total: _____				
	Fluids: oz.	Fluids: oz.	Fluids: oz.	Fluids: oz.
	Vit / Min / Supp:			

FEBRUARY 21	BREAKFAST	LUNCH	DINNER	SNACKS
S M T W T F S Carbohydrate Total per Meal: B _____ L _____ D _____ S _____ Daily Carbohydrate Total: _____				
	Fluids: oz.	Fluids: oz.	Fluids: oz.	Fluids: oz.
	Vit / Min / Supp:			

FEBRUARY 22	BREAKFAST	LUNCH	DINNER	SNACKS
S M T W T F S Carbohydrate Total per Meal: B _____ L _____ D _____ S _____ Daily Carbohydrate Total: _____				
	Fluids: oz.	Fluids: oz.	Fluids: oz.	Fluids: oz.
	Vit / Min / Supp:			

EXERCISE GOALS: _____

EXERCISE DONE: _____

FEBRUARY 23	BREAKFAST	LUNCH	DINNER	SNACKS
S M T W T F S Carbohydrate Total per Meal: B _____ L _____ D _____ S _____ Daily Carbohydrate Total: _____				
	Fluids: oz.	Fluids: oz.	Fluids: oz.	Fluids: oz.
	Vit / Min / Supp:			

FEBRUARY 24	BREAKFAST	LUNCH	DINNER	SNACKS
S M T W T F S Carbohydrate Total per Meal: B _____ L _____ D _____ S _____ Daily Carbohydrate Total: _____				
	Fluids: oz.	Fluids: oz.	Fluids: oz.	Fluids: oz.
	Vit / Min / Supp:			

FEBRUARY 25	BREAKFAST	LUNCH	DINNER	SNACKS
S M T W T F S Carbohydrate Total per Meal: B _____ L _____ D _____ S _____ Daily Carbohydrate Total: _____				
	Fluids: oz.	Fluids: oz.	Fluids: oz.	Fluids: oz.
	Vit / Min / Supp:			

TIP   Good fats are: extra-virgin, virgin, and pure olive oil as well as coconut, walnut, macadamia, hazelnut, almond, peanut, sesame seed, and avocado oils. Clarified or unsalted butter is also a good fat. Other good fat sources are coldwater fish (sardines, salmon, mackerel, herring, and tuna). Cod liver oil is a good fat, but scores low on most people's taste charts.

QUOTE   "It is good to have an end to journey towards; but it is the journey that matters, in the end." — *Ursula K. Le Guin*

GOAL FOR THE WEEK:

STATISTICS	weight	waist"	hips"
Beginning:	_____	_____	_____
End:	_____	_____	_____

FEBRUARY 26	BREAKFAST	LUNCH	DINNER	SNACKS
S M T W T F S Carbohydrate Total per Meal: B _____ L _____ D _____ S _____ Daily Carbohydrate Total: _____				
	Fluids: oz.	Fluids: oz.	Fluids: oz.	Fluids: oz.
	Vit / Min / Supp:			

FEBRUARY 27	BREAKFAST	LUNCH	DINNER	SNACKS
S M T W T F S Carbohydrate Total per Meal: B _____ L _____ D _____ S _____ Daily Carbohydrate Total: _____				
	Fluids: oz.	Fluids: oz.	Fluids: oz.	Fluids: oz.
	Vit / Min / Supp:			

FEBRUARY 28	BREAKFAST	LUNCH	DINNER	SNACKS
S M T W T F S Carbohydrate Total per Meal: B _____ L _____ D _____ S _____ Daily Carbohydrate Total: _____				
	Fluids: oz.	Fluids: oz.	Fluids: oz.	Fluids: oz.
	Vit / Min / Supp:			

FEBRUARY 29	BREAKFAST	LUNCH	DINNER	SNACKS
S M T W T F S Carbohydrate Total per Meal: B _____ L _____ D _____ S _____ Daily Carbohydrate Total: _____				
	Fluids: oz.	Fluids: oz.	Fluids: oz.	Fluids: oz.
	Vit / Min / Supp:			

EXERCISE GOALS: _____

EXERCISE DONE: _____

MARCH 1	BREAKFAST	LUNCH	DINNER	SNACKS
S M T W T F S Carbohydrate Total per Meal: B _____ L _____ D _____ S _____				
Daily Carbohydrate Total: _____	Fluids: _____ oz.	Fluids: _____ oz.	Fluids: _____ oz.	Fluids: _____ oz.
	Vit / Min / Supp:			

MARCH 2	BREAKFAST	LUNCH	DINNER	SNACKS
S M T W T F S Carbohydrate Total per Meal: B _____ L _____ D _____ S _____				
Daily Carbohydrate Total: _____	Fluids: _____ oz.	Fluids: _____ oz.	Fluids: _____ oz.	Fluids: _____ oz.
	Vit / Min / Supp:			

MARCH 3	BREAKFAST	LUNCH	DINNER	SNACKS
S M T W T F S Carbohydrate Total per Meal: B _____ L _____ D _____ S _____				
Daily Carbohydrate Total: _____	Fluids: _____ oz.	Fluids: _____ oz.	Fluids: _____ oz.	Fluids: _____ oz.
	Vit / Min / Supp:			

TIP   When you weigh and measure yourself, be brutally honest. The only person you cheat with a less than truthful answer is yourself. You deserve better than that!

QUOTE   "It only takes one person to change your life—you." — *Ruth Casey*

GOAL FOR THE WEEK:

STATISTICS	weight	waist"	hips"
Beginning:	_____	_____	_____
End:	_____	_____	_____

MARCH 4	BREAKFAST	LUNCH	DINNER	SNACKS
S M T W T F S Carbohydrate Total per Meal: B _____ L _____ D _____ S _____				
Daily Carbohydrate Total: _____	Fluids: oz.	Fluids: oz.	Fluids: oz.	Fluids: oz.
	Vit / Min / Supp:			

MARCH 5	BREAKFAST	LUNCH	DINNER	SNACKS
S M T W T F S Carbohydrate Total per Meal: B _____ L _____ D _____ S _____				
Daily Carbohydrate Total: _____	Fluids: oz.	Fluids: oz.	Fluids: oz.	Fluids: oz.
	Vit / Min / Supp:			

MARCH 6	BREAKFAST	LUNCH	DINNER	SNACKS
S M T W T F S Carbohydrate Total per Meal: B _____ L _____ D _____ S _____				
Daily Carbohydrate Total: _____	Fluids: oz.	Fluids: oz.	Fluids: oz.	Fluids: oz.
	Vit / Min / Supp:			

MARCH 7	BREAKFAST	LUNCH	DINNER	SNACKS
S M T W T F S Carbohydrate Total per Meal: B _____ L _____ D _____ S _____				
Daily Carbohydrate Total: _____	Fluids: oz.	Fluids: oz.	Fluids: oz.	Fluids: oz.
	Vit / Min / Supp:			

EXERCISE GOALS: _____

EXERCISE DONE: _____

MARCH 8	BREAKFAST	LUNCH	DINNER	SNACKS
S M T W T F S Carbohydrate Total per Meal: B _____ L _____ D _____ S _____				
Daily Carbohydrate Total: _____	Fluids: ___ oz.	Fluids: ___ oz.	Fluids: ___ oz.	Fluids: ___ oz.
	Vit / Min / Supp:			

MARCH 9	BREAKFAST	LUNCH	DINNER	SNACKS
S M T W T F S Carbohydrate Total per Meal: B _____ L _____ D _____ S _____				
Daily Carbohydrate Total: _____	Fluids: ___ oz.	Fluids: ___ oz.	Fluids: ___ oz.	Fluids: ___ oz.
	Vit / Min / Supp:			

MARCH 10	BREAKFAST	LUNCH	DINNER	SNACKS
S M T W T F S Carbohydrate Total per Meal: B _____ L _____ D _____ S _____				
Daily Carbohydrate Total: _____	Fluids: ___ oz.	Fluids: ___ oz.	Fluids: ___ oz.	Fluids: ___ oz.
	Vit / Min / Supp:			

TIP   You can interchange strawberries, blackberries, and raspberries. Each can be eaten in similar quantities, providing nearly equal carbohydrates of 3 or 4 grams per ½ cup. Boysenberries and blueberries are slightly higher at 5 to 6 grams.

QUOTE   "If the sun and moon should doubt, they'd immediately go out." — *William Blake*

GOAL FOR THE WEEK:

STATISTICS	weight	waist"	hips"
Beginning:	_____	_____	_____
End:	_____	_____	_____

165

MARCH 11	BREAKFAST	LUNCH	DINNER	SNACKS
S M T W T F S Carbohydrate Total per Meal: B _____ L _____ D _____ S _____ Daily Carbohydrate Total: _____				
	Fluids: oz.	Fluids: oz.	Fluids: oz.	Fluids: oz.
	Vit / Min / Supp:			

MARCH 12	BREAKFAST	LUNCH	DINNER	SNACKS
S M T W T F S Carbohydrate Total per Meal: B _____ L _____ D _____ S _____ Daily Carbohydrate Total: _____				
	Fluids: oz.	Fluids: oz.	Fluids: oz.	Fluids: oz.
	Vit / Min / Supp:			

MARCH 13	BREAKFAST	LUNCH	DINNER	SNACKS
S M T W T F S Carbohydrate Total per Meal: B _____ L _____ D _____ S _____ Daily Carbohydrate Total: _____				
	Fluids: oz.	Fluids: oz.	Fluids: oz.	Fluids: oz.
	Vit / Min / Supp:			

MARCH 14	BREAKFAST	LUNCH	DINNER	SNACKS
S M T W T F S Carbohydrate Total per Meal: B _____ L _____ D _____ S _____ Daily Carbohydrate Total: _____				
	Fluids: oz.	Fluids: oz.	Fluids: oz.	Fluids: oz.
	Vit / Min / Supp:			

EXERCISE GOALS: _____

EXERCISE DONE: _____

MARCH 15	BREAKFAST	LUNCH	DINNER	SNACKS
S M T W T F S Carbohydrate Total per Meal: B _____ L _____ D _____ S _____ Daily Carbohydrate Total: _____				
	Fluids: ___ oz.	Fluids: ___ oz.	Fluids: ___ oz.	Fluids: ___ oz.
	Vit / Min / Supp:			

MARCH 16	BREAKFAST	LUNCH	DINNER	SNACKS
S M T W T F S Carbohydrate Total per Meal: B _____ L _____ D _____ S _____ Daily Carbohydrate Total: _____				
	Fluids: ___ oz.	Fluids: ___ oz.	Fluids: ___ oz.	Fluids: ___ oz.
	Vit / Min / Supp:			

MARCH 17	BREAKFAST	LUNCH	DINNER	SNACKS
S M T W T F S Carbohydrate Total per Meal: B _____ L _____ D _____ S _____ Daily Carbohydrate Total: _____				
	Fluids: ___ oz.	Fluids: ___ oz.	Fluids: ___ oz.	Fluids: ___ oz.
	Vit / Min / Supp:			

TIP   Which would you rather have for 10 grams of carbohydrate: ¼ cup of cooked egg noodles or 1 cup steamed broccoli AND 1 cup sliced raw mushrooms AND 2 cups torn lettuce AND 1 oz. Roquefort dressing AND 1 sliced tomato?

QUOTE   "We all live with the objective of being happy; our lives are all different and yet the same." — *Anne Frank*

GOAL FOR THE WEEK:

STATISTICS	weight	waist"	hips"
Beginning:	_____	_____	_____
End:	_____	_____	_____

MARCH 18	BREAKFAST	LUNCH	DINNER	SNACKS
S M T W T F S Carbohydrate Total per Meal: B _____ L _____ D _____ S _____				
Daily Carbohydrate Total: _____	Fluids: _____ oz.	Fluids: _____ oz.	Fluids: _____ oz.	Fluids: _____ oz.
	Vit / Min / Supp:			

MARCH 19	BREAKFAST	LUNCH	DINNER	SNACKS
S M T W T F S Carbohydrate Total per Meal: B _____ L _____ D _____ S _____				
Daily Carbohydrate Total: _____	Fluids: _____ oz.	Fluids: _____ oz.	Fluids: _____ oz.	Fluids: _____ oz.
	Vit / Min / Supp:			

MARCH 20	BREAKFAST	LUNCH	DINNER	SNACKS
S M T W T F S Carbohydrate Total per Meal: B _____ L _____ D _____ S _____				
Daily Carbohydrate Total: _____	Fluids: _____ oz.	Fluids: _____ oz.	Fluids: _____ oz.	Fluids: _____ oz.
	Vit / Min / Supp:			

MARCH 21	BREAKFAST	LUNCH	DINNER	SNACKS
S M T W T F S Carbohydrate Total per Meal: B _____ L _____ D _____ S _____				
Daily Carbohydrate Total: _____	Fluids: _____ oz.	Fluids: _____ oz.	Fluids: _____ oz.	Fluids: _____ oz.
	Vit / Min / Supp:			

EXERCISE GOALS: _____

EXERCISE DONE: _____

168

MARCH 22	BREAKFAST	LUNCH	DINNER	SNACKS
S M T W T F S Carbohydrate Total per Meal: B _____ L _____ D _____ S _____ Daily Carbohydrate Total: _____				
	Fluids: oz.	Fluids: oz.	Fluids: oz.	Fluids: oz.
	Vit / Min / Supp:			

MARCH 23	BREAKFAST	LUNCH	DINNER	SNACKS
S M T W T F S Carbohydrate Total per Meal: B _____ L _____ D _____ S _____ Daily Carbohydrate Total: _____				
	Fluids: oz.	Fluids: oz.	Fluids: oz.	Fluids: oz.
	Vit / Min / Supp:			

MARCH 24	BREAKFAST	LUNCH	DINNER	SNACKS
S M T W T F S Carbohydrate Total per Meal: B _____ L _____ D _____ S _____ Daily Carbohydrate Total: _____				
	Fluids: oz.	Fluids: oz.	Fluids: oz.	Fluids: oz.
	Vit / Min / Supp:			

TIP   Water, water everywhere and you must surely drink your share! 64 oz. of calorie-free fluids is the daily recommendation.

QUOTE   "Without discipline, there's no life at all." — *Katharine Hepburn*

GOAL FOR THE WEEK:

STATISTICS	weight	waist"	hips"
Beginning:	_____	_____	_____
End:	_____	_____	_____

MARCH 25	BREAKFAST	LUNCH	DINNER	SNACKS
S M T W T F S Carbohydrate Total per Meal: B _____ L _____ D _____ S _____ Daily Carbohydrate Total: _____				
	Fluids: ___ oz.	Fluids: ___ oz.	Fluids: ___ oz.	Fluids: ___ oz.
	Vit / Min / Supp:			

MARCH 26	BREAKFAST	LUNCH	DINNER	SNACKS
S M T W T F S Carbohydrate Total per Meal: B _____ L _____ D _____ S _____ Daily Carbohydrate Total: _____				
	Fluids: ___ oz.	Fluids: ___ oz.	Fluids: ___ oz.	Fluids: ___ oz.
	Vit / Min / Supp:			

MARCH 27	BREAKFAST	LUNCH	DINNER	SNACKS
S M T W T F S Carbohydrate Total per Meal: B _____ L _____ D _____ S _____ Daily Carbohydrate Total: _____				
	Fluids: ___ oz.	Fluids: ___ oz.	Fluids: ___ oz.	Fluids: ___ oz.
	Vit / Min / Supp:			

MARCH 28	BREAKFAST	LUNCH	DINNER	SNACKS
S M T W T F S Carbohydrate Total per Meal: B _____ L _____ D _____ S _____ Daily Carbohydrate Total: _____				
	Fluids: ___ oz.	Fluids: ___ oz.	Fluids: ___ oz.	Fluids: ___ oz.
	Vit / Min / Supp:			

EXERCISE GOALS: _____

EXERCISE DONE: _____

MARCH 29	BREAKFAST	LUNCH	DINNER	SNACKS
S M T W T F S Carbohydrate Total per Meal: B _____ L _____ D _____ S _____ Daily Carbohydrate Total: _____				
	Fluids: _____ oz.	Fluids: _____ oz.	Fluids: _____ oz.	Fluids: _____ oz.
	Vit / Min / Supp:			

MARCH 30	BREAKFAST	LUNCH	DINNER	SNACKS
S M T W T F S Carbohydrate Total per Meal: B _____ L _____ D _____ S _____ Daily Carbohydrate Total: _____				
	Fluids: _____ oz.	Fluids: _____ oz.	Fluids: _____ oz.	Fluids: _____ oz.
	Vit / Min / Supp:			

MARCH 31	BREAKFAST	LUNCH	DINNER	SNACKS
S M T W T F S Carbohydrate Total per Meal: B _____ L _____ D _____ S _____ Daily Carbohydrate Total: _____				
	Fluids: _____ oz.	Fluids: _____ oz.	Fluids: _____ oz.	Fluids: _____ oz.
	Vit / Min / Supp:			

TIP   Punch up the flavor or food without using very many of your carbs by adding: raw chopped parsley, chopped chives, canned pimentos, raw red or white radishes, raw spinach, and raw enoki mushrooms.

QUOTE   ". . . we could never learn to be brave and patient if there were only joy in the world." — *Helen Keller*

GOAL FOR THE WEEK:

STATISTICS	weight	waist"	hips"
Beginning:	_____	_____	_____
End:	_____	_____	_____

APRIL 1	BREAKFAST	LUNCH	DINNER	SNACKS
S M T W T F S Carbohydrate Total per Meal: B _____ L _____ D _____ S _____ Daily Carbohydrate Total: _____				
	Fluids: _____ oz.	Fluids: _____ oz.	Fluids: _____ oz.	Fluids: _____ oz.
	Vit / Min / Supp:			

APRIL 2	BREAKFAST	LUNCH	DINNER	SNACKS
S M T W T F S Carbohydrate Total per Meal: B _____ L _____ D _____ S _____ Daily Carbohydrate Total: _____				
	Fluids: _____ oz.	Fluids: _____ oz.	Fluids: _____ oz.	Fluids: _____ oz.
	Vit / Min / Supp:			

APRIL 3	BREAKFAST	LUNCH	DINNER	SNACKS
S M T W T F S Carbohydrate Total per Meal: B _____ L _____ D _____ S _____ Daily Carbohydrate Total: _____				
	Fluids: _____ oz.	Fluids: _____ oz.	Fluids: _____ oz.	Fluids: _____ oz.
	Vit / Min / Supp:			

APRIL 4	BREAKFAST	LUNCH	DINNER	SNACKS
S M T W T F S Carbohydrate Total per Meal: B _____ L _____ D _____ S _____ Daily Carbohydrate Total: _____				
	Fluids: _____ oz.	Fluids: _____ oz.	Fluids: _____ oz.	Fluids: _____ oz.
	Vit / Min / Supp:			

EXERCISE GOALS: _____

EXERCISE DONE: _____

APRIL 5	BREAKFAST	LUNCH	DINNER	SNACKS
S M T W T F S Carbohydrate Total per Meal: B _____ L _____ D _____ S _____ Daily Carbohydrate Total: _____				
	Fluids: ___ oz.	Fluids: ___ oz.	Fluids: ___ oz.	Fluids: ___ oz.
	Vit / Min / Supp:			

APRIL 6	BREAKFAST	LUNCH	DINNER	SNACKS
S M T W T F S Carbohydrate Total per Meal: B _____ L _____ D _____ S _____ Daily Carbohydrate Total: _____				
	Fluids: ___ oz.	Fluids: ___ oz.	Fluids: ___ oz.	Fluids: ___ oz.
	Vit / Min / Supp:			

APRIL 7	BREAKFAST	LUNCH	DINNER	SNACKS
S M T W T F S Carbohydrate Total per Meal: B _____ L _____ D _____ S _____ Daily Carbohydrate Total: _____				
	Fluids: ___ oz.	Fluids: ___ oz.	Fluids: ___ oz.	Fluids: ___ oz.
	Vit / Min / Supp:			

TIP   One tablespoon of Parmesan or Romano cheese sprinkled on top of meats, salads, or eggs adds 2 grams of protein, 0 grams of carbohydrate, and lots of flavor.

QUOTE   "To keep a lamp burning we have to keep putting oil in it." — *Mother Teresa*

GOAL FOR THE WEEK:

STATISTICS	weight	waist"	hips"
Beginning:	_____	_____	_____
End:	_____	_____	_____

173

APRIL 8	BREAKFAST	LUNCH	DINNER	SNACKS
S M T W T F S Carbohydrate Total per Meal: B _____ L _____ D _____ S _____				
Daily Carbohydrate Total: _____	Fluids: _____ oz.	Fluids: _____ oz.	Fluids: _____ oz.	Fluids: _____ oz.
	Vit / Min / Supp:			

APRIL 9	BREAKFAST	LUNCH	DINNER	SNACKS
S M T W T F S Carbohydrate Total per Meal: B _____ L _____ D _____ S _____				
Daily Carbohydrate Total: _____	Fluids: _____ oz.	Fluids: _____ oz.	Fluids: _____ oz.	Fluids: _____ oz.
	Vit / Min / Supp:			

APRIL 10	BREAKFAST	LUNCH	DINNER	SNACKS
S M T W T F S Carbohydrate Total per Meal: B _____ L _____ D _____ S _____				
Daily Carbohydrate Total: _____	Fluids: _____ oz.	Fluids: _____ oz.	Fluids: _____ oz.	Fluids: _____ oz.
	Vit / Min / Supp:			

APRIL 11	BREAKFAST	LUNCH	DINNER	SNACKS
S M T W T F S Carbohydrate Total per Meal: B _____ L _____ D _____ S _____				
Daily Carbohydrate Total: _____	Fluids: _____ oz.	Fluids: _____ oz.	Fluids: _____ oz.	Fluids: _____ oz.
	Vit / Min / Supp:			

EXERCISE GOALS: _____

EXERCISE DONE: _____

174

APRIL 12	BREAKFAST	LUNCH	DINNER	SNACKS
S M T W T F S Carbohydrate Total per Meal: B _____ L _____ D _____ S _____				
Daily Carbohydrate Total: _____	Fluids: oz.	Fluids: oz.	Fluids: oz.	Fluids: oz.
	Vit / Min / Supp:			

APRIL 13	BREAKFAST	LUNCH	DINNER	SNACKS
S M T W T F S Carbohydrate Total per Meal: B _____ L _____ D _____ S _____				
Daily Carbohydrate Total: _____	Fluids: oz.	Fluids: oz.	Fluids: oz.	Fluids: oz.
	Vit / Min / Supp:			

APRIL 14	BREAKFAST	LUNCH	DINNER	SNACKS
S M T W T F S Carbohydrate Total per Meal: B _____ L _____ D _____ S _____				
Daily Carbohydrate Total: _____	Fluids: oz.	Fluids: oz.	Fluids: oz.	Fluids: oz.
	Vit / Min / Supp:			

TIP   Create a Protein Power tea party for your afternoon snack. Prepare a pot of nice hot tea. Serve slices of cucumber topped with Neufchatel cheese and deli slices of turkey along with roll-ups made with Neufchatel cheese and Dijon mustard spread on slices of non-sugar-cured ham and rolled around a green onion; add salt and white pepper to taste. Each guest receives two cucumber canapés and one roll-up with unlimited cups of tea with or without a bit of milk. For a festive touch, serve two strawberries to garnish each plate.

QUOTE   "The mind grows by what it feeds on." — *Josiah G. Holland*

GOAL FOR THE WEEK:

STATISTICS	weight	waist"	hips"
Beginning:	_____	_____	_____
End:	_____	_____	_____

APRIL 15	BREAKFAST	LUNCH	DINNER	SNACKS
S M T W T F S Carbohydrate Total per Meal: B _____ L _____ D _____ S _____				
Daily Carbohydrate Total: _____	Fluids: oz.	Fluids: oz.	Fluids: oz.	Fluids: oz.
	Vit / Min / Supp:			

APRIL 16	BREAKFAST	LUNCH	DINNER	SNACKS
S M T W T F S Carbohydrate Total per Meal: B _____ L _____ D _____ S _____				
Daily Carbohydrate Total: _____	Fluids: oz.	Fluids: oz.	Fluids: oz.	Fluids: oz.
	Vit / Min / Supp:			

APRIL 17	BREAKFAST	LUNCH	DINNER	SNACKS
S M T W T F S Carbohydrate Total per Meal: B _____ L _____ D _____ S _____				
Daily Carbohydrate Total: _____	Fluids: oz.	Fluids: oz.	Fluids: oz.	Fluids: oz.
	Vit / Min / Supp:			

APRIL 18	BREAKFAST	LUNCH	DINNER	SNACKS
S M T W T F S Carbohydrate Total per Meal: B _____ L _____ D _____ S _____				
Daily Carbohydrate Total: _____	Fluids: oz.	Fluids: oz.	Fluids: oz.	Fluids: oz.
	Vit / Min / Supp:			

EXERCISE GOALS: _____

EXERCISE DONE: _____

APRIL 19	BREAKFAST	LUNCH	DINNER	SNACKS
S M T W T F S Carbohydrate Total per Meal: B _____ L _____ D _____ S _____				
Daily Carbohydrate Total: _____	Fluids: oz.	Fluids: oz.	Fluids: oz.	Fluids: oz.
	Vit / Min / Supp:			

APRIL 20	BREAKFAST	LUNCH	DINNER	SNACKS
S M T W T F S Carbohydrate Total per Meal: B _____ L _____ D _____ S _____				.
Daily Carbohydrate Total: _____	Fluids: oz.	Fluids: oz.	Fluids: oz.	Fluids: oz.
	Vit / Min / Supp:			

APRIL 21	BREAKFAST	LUNCH	DINNER	SNACKS
S M T W T F S Carbohydrate Total per Meal: B _____ L _____ D _____ S _____				
Daily Carbohydrate Total: _____	Fluids: oz.	Fluids: oz.	Fluids: oz.	Fluids: oz.
	Vit / Min / Supp:			

TIP   In addition to your good diet, take a good vitamin and mineral supplement—every day.

QUOTE   "Argue for your limitations, and sure enough, they're yours." — *Richard Bach*

GOAL FOR THE WEEK:

STATISTICS	weight	waist"	hips"
Beginning:	_____	_____	_____
End:	_____	_____	_____

177

APRIL 22 S M T W T F S Carbohydrate Total per Meal: B _____ L _____ D _____ S _____ Daily Carbohydrate Total: _____	**BREAKFAST**	**LUNCH**	**DINNER**	**SNACKS**
	Fluids: oz.	Fluids: oz.	Fluids: oz.	Fluids: oz.
	Vit / Min / Supp:			

APRIL 23 S M T W T F S Carbohydrate Total per Meal: B _____ L _____ D _____ S _____ Daily Carbohydrate Total: _____	**BREAKFAST**	**LUNCH**	**DINNER**	**SNACKS**
	Fluids: oz.	Fluids: oz.	Fluids: oz.	Fluids: oz.
	Vit / Min / Supp:			

APRIL 24 S M T W T F S Carbohydrate Total per Meal: B _____ L _____ D _____ S _____ Daily Carbohydrate Total: _____	**BREAKFAST**	**LUNCH**	**DINNER**	**SNACKS**
	Fluids: oz.	Fluids: oz.	Fluids: oz.	Fluids: oz.
	Vit / Min / Supp:			

APRIL 25 S M T W T F S Carbohydrate Total per Meal: B _____ L _____ D _____ S _____ Daily Carbohydrate Total: _____	**BREAKFAST**	**LUNCH**	**DINNER**	**SNACKS**
	Fluids: oz.	Fluids: oz.	Fluids: oz.	Fluids: oz.
	Vit / Min / Supp:			

EXERCISE GOALS: _____

EXERCISE DONE: _____

APRIL 26	BREAKFAST	LUNCH	DINNER	SNACKS
S M T W T F S Carbohydrate Total per Meal: B _____ L _____ D _____ S _____				
Daily Carbohydrate Total: _____	Fluids: _____ oz.	Fluids: _____ oz.	Fluids: _____ oz.	Fluids: _____ oz.
	Vit / Min / Supp:			

APRIL 27	BREAKFAST	LUNCH	DINNER	SNACKS
S M T W T F S Carbohydrate Total per Meal: B _____ L _____ D _____ S _____				
Daily Carbohydrate Total: _____	Fluids: _____ oz.	Fluids: _____ oz.	Fluids: _____ oz.	Fluids: _____ oz.
	Vit / Min / Supp:			

APRIL 28	BREAKFAST	LUNCH	DINNER	SNACKS
S M T W T F S Carbohydrate Total per Meal: B _____ L _____ D _____ S _____				
Daily Carbohydrate Total: _____	Fluids: _____ oz.	Fluids: _____ oz.	Fluids: _____ oz.	Fluids: _____ oz.
	Vit / Min / Supp:			

TIP   Experiment! For a breakfast taste treat try one whole egg and two egg whites scrambled with smoked salmon and dill or cottage cheese and chives or grated Gruyere and fresh asparagus tips.

QUOTE   "You grow up the day you have the first real laugh—at yourself!" — *Ethel Barrymore*

GOAL FOR THE WEEK:

STATISTICS	weight	waist"	hips"
Beginning:	_____	_____	_____
End:	_____	_____	_____

179

APRIL 29	BREAKFAST	LUNCH	DINNER	SNACKS
S M T W T F S Carbohydrate Total per Meal: B _____ L _____ D _____ S _____ Daily Carbohydrate Total: _____				
	Fluids: oz.	Fluids: oz.	Fluids: oz.	Fluids: oz.
	Vit / Min / Supp:			

APRIL 30	BREAKFAST	LUNCH	DINNER	SNACKS
S M T W T F S Carbohydrate Total per Meal: B _____ L _____ D _____ S _____ Daily Carbohydrate Total: _____				
	Fluids: oz.	Fluids: oz.	Fluids: oz.	Fluids: oz.
	Vit / Min / Supp:			

MAY 1	BREAKFAST	LUNCH	DINNER	SNACKS
S M T W T F S Carbohydrate Total per Meal: B _____ L _____ D _____ S _____ Daily Carbohydrate Total: _____				
	Fluids: oz.	Fluids: oz.	Fluids: oz.	Fluids: oz.
	Vit / Min / Supp:			

MAY 2	BREAKFAST	LUNCH	DINNER	SNACKS
S M T W T F S Carbohydrate Total per Meal: B _____ L _____ D _____ S _____ Daily Carbohydrate Total: _____				
	Fluids: oz.	Fluids: oz.	Fluids: oz.	Fluids: oz.
	Vit / Min / Supp:			

EXERCISE GOALS: _____

EXERCISE DONE: _____

MAY 3	BREAKFAST	LUNCH	DINNER	SNACKS
S M T W T F S Carbohydrate Total per Meal: B _____ L _____ D _____ S _____				
Daily Carbohydrate Total: _____	Fluids: oz.	Fluids: oz.	Fluids: oz.	Fluids: oz.
	Vit / Min / Supp:			

MAY 4	BREAKFAST	LUNCH	DINNER	SNACKS
S M T W T F S Carbohydrate Total per Meal: B _____ L _____ D _____ S _____				
Daily Carbohydrate Total: _____	Fluids: oz.	Fluids: oz.	Fluids: oz.	Fluids: oz.
	Vit / Min / Supp:			

MAY 5	BREAKFAST	LUNCH	DINNER	SNACKS
S M T W T F S Carbohydrate Total per Meal: B _____ L _____ D _____ S _____				
Daily Carbohydrate Total: _____	Fluids: oz.	Fluids: oz.	Fluids: oz.	Fluids: oz.
	Vit / Min / Supp:			

TIP   Dress up your coffee without adding carbs. Add ½ teaspoon ground cardamom seed and ½ teaspoon ground cinnamon to enough ground coffee for eight cups—then brew or press. The aroma is as delightful as the flavor.

QUOTE   "Human beings, by changing the inner attitudes of their minds, can change the outer aspects of their lives." — William James

GOAL FOR THE WEEK:

STATISTICS	weight	waist"	hips"
Beginning:	_____	_____	_____
End:	_____	_____	_____

MAY 6	BREAKFAST	LUNCH	DINNER	SNACKS
S M T W T F S Carbohydrate Total per Meal: B _____ L _____ D _____ S _____ Daily Carbohydrate Total: _____				
	Fluids: _____ oz.	Fluids: _____ oz.	Fluids: _____ oz.	Fluids: _____ oz.
	Vit / Min / Supp:			

MAY 7	BREAKFAST	LUNCH	DINNER	SNACKS
S M T W T F S Carbohydrate Total per Meal: B _____ L _____ D _____ S _____ Daily Carbohydrate Total: _____				
	Fluids: _____ oz.	Fluids: _____ oz.	Fluids: _____ oz.	Fluids: _____ oz.
	Vit / Min / Supp:			

MAY 8	BREAKFAST	LUNCH	DINNER	SNACKS
S M T W T F S Carbohydrate Total per Meal: B _____ L _____ D _____ S _____ Daily Carbohydrate Total: _____				
	Fluids: _____ oz.	Fluids: _____ oz.	Fluids: _____ oz.	Fluids: _____ oz.
	Vit / Min / Supp:			

MAY 9	BREAKFAST	LUNCH	DINNER	SNACKS
S M T W T F S Carbohydrate Total per Meal: B _____ L _____ D _____ S _____ Daily Carbohydrate Total: _____				
	Fluids: _____ oz.	Fluids: _____ oz.	Fluids: _____ oz.	Fluids: _____ oz.
	Vit / Min / Supp:			

EXERCISE GOALS: _____

EXERCISE DONE: _____

MAY 10	BREAKFAST	LUNCH	DINNER	SNACKS
S M T W T F S Carbohydrate Total per Meal: B _____ L _____ D _____ S _____				
Daily Carbohydrate Total: _____	Fluids: ____ oz.	Fluids: ____ oz.	Fluids: ____ oz.	Fluids: ____ oz.
	Vit / Min / Supp:			

MAY 11	BREAKFAST	LUNCH	DINNER	SNACKS
S M T W T F S Carbohydrate Total per Meal: B _____ L _____ D _____ S _____				
Daily Carbohydrate Total: _____	Fluids: ____ oz.	Fluids: ____ oz.	Fluids: ____ oz.	Fluids: ____ oz.
	Vit / Min / Supp:			

MAY 12	BREAKFAST	LUNCH	DINNER	SNACKS
S M T W T F S Carbohydrate Total per Meal: B _____ L _____ D _____ S _____				
Daily Carbohydrate Total: _____	Fluids: ____ oz.	Fluids: ____ oz.	Fluids: ____ oz.	Fluids: ____ oz.
	Vit / Min / Supp:			

TIP   Remember, the body understands that protein is its most critical nutrient. And the body keys its metabolic rate (the number of calories it uses each day) to the amount of incoming protein it receives.

QUOTE   "Experience is not what happens to you, it is what you do with what happens to you." — *Aldous Huxley*

GOAL FOR THE WEEK:

STATISTICS	weight	waist"	hips"
Beginning:	_____	_____	_____
End:	_____	_____	_____

MAY 13	BREAKFAST	LUNCH	DINNER	SNACKS
S M T W T F S Carbohydrate Total per Meal: B _____ L _____ D _____ S _____ Daily Carbohydrate Total: _____				
	Fluids: _____ oz.	Fluids: _____ oz.	Fluids: _____ oz.	Fluids: _____ oz.
	Vit / Min / Supp:			

MAY 14	BREAKFAST	LUNCH	DINNER	SNACKS
S M T W T F S Carbohydrate Total per Meal: B _____ L _____ D _____ S _____ Daily Carbohydrate Total: _____				
	Fluids: _____ oz.	Fluids: _____ oz.	Fluids: _____ oz.	Fluids: _____ oz.
	Vit / Min / Supp:			

MAY 15	BREAKFAST	LUNCH	DINNER	SNACKS
S M T W T F S Carbohydrate Total per Meal: B _____ L _____ D _____ S _____ Daily Carbohydrate Total: _____				
	Fluids: _____ oz.	Fluids: _____ oz.	Fluids: _____ oz.	Fluids: _____ oz.
	Vit / Min / Supp:			

MAY 16	BREAKFAST	LUNCH	DINNER	SNACKS
S M T W T F S Carbohydrate Total per Meal: B _____ L _____ D _____ S _____ Daily Carbohydrate Total: _____				
	Fluids: _____ oz.	Fluids: _____ oz.	Fluids: _____ oz.	Fluids: _____ oz.
	Vit / Min / Supp:			

EXERCISE GOALS: _____

EXERCISE DONE: _____

184

MAY 17	BREAKFAST	LUNCH	DINNER	SNACKS
S M T W T F S Carbohydrate Total per Meal: B _____ L _____ D _____ S _____ Daily Carbohydrate Total: _____				
	Fluids: oz.	Fluids: oz.	Fluids: oz.	Fluids: oz.
	Vit / Min / Supp:			

MAY 18	BREAKFAST	LUNCH	DINNER	SNACKS
S M T W T F S Carbohydrate Total per Meal: B _____ L _____ D _____ S _____ Daily Carbohydrate Total: _____				
	Fluids: oz.	Fluids: oz.	Fluids: oz.	Fluids: oz.
	Vit / Min / Supp:			

MAY 19	BREAKFAST	LUNCH	DINNER	SNACKS
S M T W T F S Carbohydrate Total per Meal: B _____ L _____ D _____ S _____ Daily Carbohydrate Total: _____				
	Fluids: oz.	Fluids: oz.	Fluids: oz.	Fluids: oz.
	Vit / Min / Supp:			

TIP   Your daily requirement for carbohydrate is ZERO! That's right—none, nada, zippo! Your body—actually your liver—has the ability to take dietary protein or fat (or your own body fat) and make glucose from it.

QUOTE   "Courage faces fear and thereby masters it." — *Martin Luther King Jr.*

GOAL FOR THE WEEK:

STATISTICS	weight	waist"	hips"
Beginning:	_____	_____	_____
End:	_____	_____	_____

MAY 20	BREAKFAST	LUNCH	DINNER	SNACKS
S M T W T F S Carbohydrate Total per Meal: B _____ L _____ D _____ S _____ Daily Carbohydrate Total: _____				
	Fluids: oz.	Fluids: oz.	Fluids: oz.	Fluids: oz.
	Vit / Min / Supp:			

MAY 21	BREAKFAST	LUNCH	DINNER	SNACKS
S M T W T F S Carbohydrate Total per Meal: B _____ L _____ D _____ S _____ Daily Carbohydrate Total: _____				
	Fluids: oz.	Fluids: oz.	Fluids: oz.	Fluids: oz.
	Vit / Min / Supp:			

MAY 22	BREAKFAST	LUNCH	DINNER	SNACKS
S M T W T F S Carbohydrate Total per Meal: B _____ L _____ D _____ S _____ Daily Carbohydrate Total: _____				
	Fluids: oz.	Fluids: oz.	Fluids: oz.	Fluids: oz.
	Vit / Min / Supp:			

MAY 23	BREAKFAST	LUNCH	DINNER	SNACKS
S M T W T F S Carbohydrate Total per Meal: B _____ L _____ D _____ S _____ Daily Carbohydrate Total: _____				
	Fluids: oz.	Fluids: oz.	Fluids: oz.	Fluids: oz.
	Vit / Min / Supp:			

EXERCISE GOALS: _____

EXERCISE DONE: _____

MAY 24	BREAKFAST	LUNCH	DINNER	SNACKS
S M T W T F S Carbohydrate Total per Meal: B _____ L _____ D _____ S _____ Daily Carbohydrate Total: _____				
	Fluids: ____ oz.	Fluids: ____ oz.	Fluids: ____ oz.	Fluids: ____ oz.
	Vit / Min / Supp:			

MAY 25	BREAKFAST	LUNCH	DINNER	SNACKS
S M T W T F S Carbohydrate Total per Meal: B _____ L _____ D _____ S _____ Daily Carbohydrate Total: _____				
	Fluids: ____ oz.	Fluids: ____ oz.	Fluids: ____ oz.	Fluids: ____ oz.
	Vit / Min / Supp:			

MAY 26	BREAKFAST	LUNCH	DINNER	SNACKS
S M T W T F S Carbohydrate Total per Meal: B _____ L _____ D _____ S _____ Daily Carbohydrate Total: _____				
	Fluids: ____ oz.	Fluids: ____ oz.	Fluids: ____ oz.	Fluids: ____ oz.
	Vit / Min / Supp:			

TIP   No food is free—there's a metabolic consequence to every bite you eat. It may be a good one, or it may be a disastrous one, but one thing is certain: when you eat, something is going to happen. Your choice determines whether it is good or not.

QUOTE   "Be not afraid of growing slowly, be afraid only of standing still." — *Chinese proverb*

GOAL FOR THE WEEK:

STATISTICS	weight	waist"	hips"
Beginning:	_____	_____	_____
End:	_____	_____	_____

MAY 27	BREAKFAST	LUNCH	DINNER	SNACKS
S M T W T F S Carbohydrate Total per Meal: B _____ L _____ D _____ S _____ Daily Carbohydrate Total: _____				
	Fluids: oz.	Fluids: oz.	Fluids: oz.	Fluids: oz.
	Vit / Min / Supp:			

MAY 28	BREAKFAST	LUNCH	DINNER	SNACKS
S M T W T F S Carbohydrate Total per Meal: B _____ L _____ D _____ S _____ Daily Carbohydrate Total: _____				
	Fluids: oz.	Fluids: oz.	Fluids: oz.	Fluids: oz.
	Vit / Min / Supp:			

MAY 29	BREAKFAST	LUNCH	DINNER	SNACKS
S M T W T F S Carbohydrate Total per Meal: B _____ L _____ D _____ S _____ Daily Carbohydrate Total: _____				
	Fluids: oz.	Fluids: oz.	Fluids: oz.	Fluids: oz.
	Vit / Min / Supp:			

MAY 30	BREAKFAST	LUNCH	DINNER	SNACKS
S M T W T F S Carbohydrate Total per Meal: B _____ L _____ D _____ S _____ Daily Carbohydrate Total: _____				
	Fluids: oz.	Fluids: oz.	Fluids: oz.	Fluids: oz.
	Vit / Min / Supp:			

EXERCISE GOALS: _____

EXERCISE DONE: _____

MAY 31	BREAKFAST	LUNCH	DINNER	SNACKS
S M T W T F S Carbohydrate Total per Meal: B _____ L _____ D _____ S _____ Daily Carbohydrate Total: _____				
	Fluids: ___ oz.	Fluids: ___ oz.	Fluids: ___ oz.	Fluids: ___ oz.
	Vit / Min / Supp:			

JUNE 1	BREAKFAST	LUNCH	DINNER	SNACKS
S M T W T F S Carbohydrate Total per Meal: B _____ L _____ D _____ S _____ Daily Carbohydrate Total: _____				
	Fluids: ___ oz.	Fluids: ___ oz.	Fluids: ___ oz.	Fluids: ___ oz.
	Vit / Min / Supp:			

JUNE 2	BREAKFAST	LUNCH	DINNER	SNACKS
S M T W T F S Carbohydrate Total per Meal: B _____ L _____ D _____ S _____ Daily Carbohydrate Total: _____				
	Fluids: ___ oz.	Fluids: ___ oz.	Fluids: ___ oz.	Fluids: ___ oz.
	Vit / Min / Supp:			

TIP   Treat yourself well visually—use a very attractive glass for your calorie-free fluids and add a very thin slice of lemon or lime to your water.

QUOTE   "Self-discipline is self-caring." — M. Scott Peck

GOAL FOR THE WEEK:

STATISTICS	weight	waist"	hips"
Beginning:	_____	_____	_____
End:	_____	_____	_____

JUNE 3	BREAKFAST	LUNCH	DINNER	SNACKS
S M T W T F S Carbohydrate Total per Meal: B _____ L _____ D _____ S _____				
Daily Carbohydrate Total: _____	Fluids: oz.	Fluids: oz.	Fluids: oz.	Fluids: oz.
	Vit / Min / Supp:			

JUNE 4	BREAKFAST	LUNCH	DINNER	SNACKS
S M T W T F S Carbohydrate Total per Meal: B _____ L _____ D _____ S _____				
Daily Carbohydrate Total: _____	Fluids: oz.	Fluids: oz.	Fluids: oz.	Fluids: oz.
	Vit / Min / Supp:			

JUNE 5	BREAKFAST	LUNCH	DINNER	SNACKS
S M T W T F S Carbohydrate Total per Meal: B _____ L _____ D _____ S _____				
Daily Carbohydrate Total: _____	Fluids: oz.	Fluids: oz.	Fluids: oz.	Fluids: oz.
	Vit / Min / Supp:			

JUNE 6	BREAKFAST	LUNCH	DINNER	SNACKS
S M T W T F S Carbohydrate Total per Meal: B _____ L _____ D _____ S _____				
Daily Carbohydrate Total: _____	Fluids: oz.	Fluids: oz.	Fluids: oz.	Fluids: oz.
	Vit / Min / Supp:			

EXERCISE GOALS: _____

EXERCISE DONE: _____

JUNE 7	BREAKFAST	LUNCH	DINNER	SNACKS
S M T W T F S Carbohydrate Total per Meal: B _____ L _____ D _____ S _____				
Daily Carbohydrate Total: _____	Fluids: oz.	Fluids: oz.	Fluids: oz.	Fluids: oz.
	Vit / Min / Supp:			

JUNE 8	BREAKFAST	LUNCH	DINNER	SNACKS
S M T W T F S Carbohydrate Total per Meal: B _____ L _____ D _____ S _____				
Daily Carbohydrate Total: _____	Fluids: oz.	Fluids: oz.	Fluids: oz.	Fluids: oz.
	Vit / Min / Supp:			

JUNE 9	BREAKFAST	LUNCH	DINNER	SNACKS
S M T W T F S Carbohydrate Total per Meal: B _____ L _____ D _____ S _____				
Daily Carbohydrate Total: _____	Fluids: oz.	Fluids: oz.	Fluids: oz.	Fluids: oz.
	Vit / Min / Supp:			

TIP   Give yourself an extra nudge. Park your vehicle at the far corner of all parking lots and hike to your destination. As often as possible, use stairs rather than an elevator. If you're going to the thirty-seventh floor, get off on thirty-two and walk the rest of the way.

QUOTE   "As long as you live, keep learning how to live." — *Seneca*

GOAL FOR THE WEEK:

STATISTICS	weight	waist"	hips"
Beginning:	_____	_____	_____
End:	_____	_____	_____

JUNE 10	BREAKFAST	LUNCH	DINNER	SNACKS
S M T W T F S Carbohydrate Total per Meal: B _____ L _____ D _____ S _____				
Daily Carbohydrate Total: _____	Fluids: _____ oz.	Fluids: _____ oz.	Fluids: _____ oz.	Fluids: _____ oz.
	Vit / Min / Supp:			

JUNE 11	BREAKFAST	LUNCH	DINNER	SNACKS
S M T W T F S Carbohydrate Total per Meal: B _____ L _____ D _____ S _____				
Daily Carbohydrate Total: _____	Fluids: _____ oz.	Fluids: _____ oz.	Fluids: _____ oz.	Fluids: _____ oz.
	Vit / Min / Supp:			

JUNE 12	BREAKFAST	LUNCH	DINNER	SNACKS
S M T W T F S Carbohydrate Total per Meal: B _____ L _____ D _____ S _____				
Daily Carbohydrate Total: _____	Fluids: _____ oz.	Fluids: _____ oz.	Fluids: _____ oz.	Fluids: _____ oz.
	Vit / Min / Supp:			

JUNE 13	BREAKFAST	LUNCH	DINNER	SNACKS
S M T W T F S Carbohydrate Total per Meal: B _____ L _____ D _____ S _____				
Daily Carbohydrate Total: _____	Fluids: _____ oz.	Fluids: _____ oz.	Fluids: _____ oz.	Fluids: _____ oz.
	Vit / Min / Supp:			

EXERCISE GOALS: _____

EXERCISE DONE: _____

JUNE 14	BREAKFAST	LUNCH	DINNER	SNACKS
S M T W T F S Carbohydrate Total per Meal: B _____ L _____ D _____ S _____				
Daily Carbohydrate Total: _____	Fluids: _____ oz.	Fluids: _____ oz.	Fluids: _____ oz.	Fluids: _____ oz.
	Vit/Min/Supp:			

JUNE 15	BREAKFAST	LUNCH	DINNER	SNACKS
S M T W T F S Carbohydrate Total per Meal: B _____ L _____ D _____ S _____				
Daily Carbohydrate Total: _____	Fluids: _____ oz.	Fluids: _____ oz.	Fluids: _____ oz.	Fluids: _____ oz.
	Vit/Min/Supp:			

JUNE 16	BREAKFAST	LUNCH	DINNER	SNACKS
S M T W T F S Carbohydrate Total per Meal: B _____ L _____ D _____ S _____				
Daily Carbohydrate Total: _____	Fluids: _____ oz.	Fluids: _____ oz.	Fluids: _____ oz.	Fluids: _____ oz.
	Vit/Min/Supp:			

TIP   Plan a weekly date with yourself that has nothing to do with food. Visit a museum, go to a concert, take in a movie, volunteer at a hospital or school in your community, take a long walk, plant some flowers or herbs, but make the activity something you do not do routinely.

QUOTE   "The human mind always makes progress, but it is a progress in spirals." — *Madame de Staël*

GOAL FOR THE WEEK:

STATISTICS	weight	waist"	hips"
Beginning:	_____	_____	_____
End:	_____	_____	_____

JUNE 17	BREAKFAST	LUNCH	DINNER	SNACKS
S M T W T F S Carbohydrate Total per Meal: B _____ L _____ D _____ S _____ Daily Carbohydrate Total: _____				
	Fluids: _____ oz.	Fluids: _____ oz.	Fluids: _____ oz.	Fluids: _____ oz.
	Vit / Min / Supp:			

JUNE 18	BREAKFAST	LUNCH	DINNER	SNACKS
S M T W T F S Carbohydrate Total per Meal: B _____ L _____ D _____ S _____ Daily Carbohydrate Total: _____				
	Fluids: _____ oz.	Fluids: _____ oz.	Fluids: _____ oz.	Fluids: _____ oz.
	Vit / Min / Supp:			

JUNE 19	BREAKFAST	LUNCH	DINNER	SNACKS
S M T W T F S Carbohydrate Total per Meal: B _____ L _____ D _____ S _____ Daily Carbohydrate Total: _____				
	Fluids: _____ oz.	Fluids: _____ oz.	Fluids: _____ oz.	Fluids: _____ oz.
	Vit / Min / Supp:			

JUNE 20	BREAKFAST	LUNCH	DINNER	SNACKS
S M T W T F S Carbohydrate Total per Meal: B _____ L _____ D _____ S _____ Daily Carbohydrate Total: _____				
	Fluids: _____ oz.	Fluids: _____ oz.	Fluids: _____ oz.	Fluids: _____ oz.
	Vit / Min / Supp:			

EXERCISE GOALS: _____

EXERCISE DONE: _____

JUNE 21	BREAKFAST	LUNCH	DINNER	SNACKS
S M T W T F S Carbohydrate Total per Meal: B _____ L _____ D _____ S _____				
Daily Carbohydrate Total: _____	Fluids: oz.	Fluids: oz.	Fluids: oz.	Fluids: oz.
	Vit / Min / Supp:			

JUNE 22	BREAKFAST	LUNCH	DINNER	SNACKS
S M T W T F S Carbohydrate Total per Meal: B _____ L _____ D _____ S _____				
Daily Carbohydrate Total: _____	Fluids: oz.	Fluids: oz.	Fluids: oz.	Fluids: oz.
	Vit / Min / Supp:			

JUNE 23	BREAKFAST	LUNCH	DINNER	SNACKS
S M T W T F S Carbohydrate Total per Meal: B _____ L _____ D _____ S _____				
Daily Carbohydrate Total: _____	Fluids: oz.	Fluids: oz.	Fluids: oz.	Fluids: oz.
	Vit / Min / Supp:			

TIP   Even a non-gardener can plant a salad pot. Scout out several varieties of leaf lettuce that will grow in your climate. Use a large pot placed in a sunny location and sow all the types of lettuce together. Keep the soil moist, and soon you will be harvesting your own fresh salad greens.

QUOTE   "I find the great thing in this world is not so much where we stand as in what direction we are moving."
— Oliver Wendell Holmes

GOAL FOR THE WEEK:

STATISTICS	weight	waist"	hips"
Beginning:	_____	_____	_____
End:	_____	_____	_____

JUNE 24	BREAKFAST	LUNCH	DINNER	SNACKS
S M T W T F S Carbohydrate Total per Meal: B _____ L _____ D _____ S _____ Daily Carbohydrate Total: _____				
	Fluids: oz.	Fluids: oz.	Fluids: oz.	Fluids: oz.
	Vit / Min / Supp:			

JUNE 25	BREAKFAST	LUNCH	DINNER	SNACKS
S M T W T F S Carbohydrate Total per Meal: B _____ L _____ D _____ S _____ Daily Carbohydrate Total: _____				
	Fluids: oz.	Fluids: oz.	Fluids: oz.	Fluids: oz.
	Vit / Min / Supp:			

JUNE 26	BREAKFAST	LUNCH	DINNER	SNACKS
S M T W T F S Carbohydrate Total per Meal: B _____ L _____ D _____ S _____ Daily Carbohydrate Total: _____				
	Fluids: oz.	Fluids: oz.	Fluids: oz.	Fluids: oz.
	Vit / Min / Supp:			

JUNE 27	BREAKFAST	LUNCH	DINNER	SNACKS
S M T W T F S Carbohydrate Total per Meal: B _____ L _____ D _____ S _____ Daily Carbohydrate Total: _____				
	Fluids: oz.	Fluids: oz.	Fluids: oz.	Fluids: oz.
	Vit / Min / Supp:			

EXERCISE GOALS: _____

EXERCISE DONE: _____

JUNE 28	BREAKFAST	LUNCH	DINNER	SNACKS
S M T W T F S Carbohydrate Total per Meal: B _____ L _____ D _____ S _____ Daily Carbohydrate Total: _____				
	Fluids: _____ oz.	Fluids: _____ oz.	Fluids: _____ oz.	Fluids: _____ oz.
	Vit / Min / Supp:			

JUNE 29	BREAKFAST	LUNCH	DINNER	SNACKS
S M T W T F S Carbohydrate Total per Meal: B _____ L _____ D _____ S _____ Daily Carbohydrate Total: _____				
	Fluids: _____ oz.	Fluids: _____ oz.	Fluids: _____ oz.	Fluids: _____ oz.
	Vit / Min / Supp:			

JUNE 30	BREAKFAST	LUNCH	DINNER	SNACKS
S M T W T F S Carbohydrate Total per Meal: B _____ L _____ D _____ S _____ Daily Carbohydrate Total: _____				
	Fluids: _____ oz.	Fluids: _____ oz.	Fluids: _____ oz.	Fluids: _____ oz.
	Vit / Min / Supp:			

TIP   During favorable weather pack your Staying Power lunch (or any other meal) and escape to a park for a special treat. You will not be tempted to eat something you should not and you'll save money as well.

QUOTE   "All glory comes from daring to begin." — *Eugene F. Ware*

GOAL FOR THE WEEK:

STATISTICS	weight	waist"	hips"
Beginning:	_____	_____	_____
End:	_____	_____	_____

JULY 1	BREAKFAST	LUNCH	DINNER	SNACKS
S M T W T F S Carbohydrate Total per Meal: B _____ L _____ D _____ S _____				
Daily Carbohydrate Total: _____	Fluids: ____ oz.	Fluids: ____ oz.	Fluids: ____ oz.	Fluids: ____ oz.
	Vit / Min / Supp:			

JULY 2	BREAKFAST	LUNCH	DINNER	SNACKS
S M T W T F S Carbohydrate Total per Meal: B _____ L _____ D _____ S _____				
Daily Carbohydrate Total: _____	Fluids: ____ oz.	Fluids: ____ oz.	Fluids: ____ oz.	Fluids: ____ oz.
	Vit / Min / Supp:			

JULY 3	BREAKFAST	LUNCH	DINNER	SNACKS
S M T W T F S Carbohydrate Total per Meal: B _____ L _____ D _____ S _____				
Daily Carbohydrate Total: _____	Fluids: ____ oz.	Fluids: ____ oz.	Fluids: ____ oz.	Fluids: ____ oz.
	Vit / Min / Supp:			

JULY 4	BREAKFAST	LUNCH	DINNER	SNACKS
S M T W T F S Carbohydrate Total per Meal: B _____ L _____ D _____ S _____				
Daily Carbohydrate Total: _____	Fluids: ____ oz.	Fluids: ____ oz.	Fluids: ____ oz.	Fluids: ____ oz.
	Vit / Min / Supp:			

EXERCISE GOALS: _____

EXERCISE DONE: _____

198

JULY 5	BREAKFAST	LUNCH	DINNER	SNACKS
S M T W T F S Carbohydrate Total per Meal: B _____ L _____ D _____ S _____ Daily Carbohydrate Total: _____				
	Fluids: oz.	Fluids: oz.	Fluids: oz.	Fluids: oz.
	Vit / Min / Supp:			

JULY 6	BREAKFAST	LUNCH	DINNER	SNACKS
S M T W T F S Carbohydrate Total per Meal: B _____ L _____ D _____ S _____ Daily Carbohydrate Total: _____				
	Fluids: oz.	Fluids: oz.	Fluids: oz.	Fluids: oz.
	Vit / Min / Supp:			

JULY 7	BREAKFAST	LUNCH	DINNER	SNACKS
S M T W T F S Carbohydrate Total per Meal: B _____ L _____ D _____ S _____ Daily Carbohydrate Total: _____				
	Fluids: oz.	Fluids: oz.	Fluids: oz.	Fluids: oz.
	Vit / Min / Supp:			

TIP   Eating out selections to avoid: bread or rolls, potatoes, sugary desserts, pasta dishes, steamed or fried rice, noodles, breaded items, bread sticks, sweet wines, pizza crust, and sandwich buns. Instead of potatoes, rice, or pasta, ask the waiter to substitute a serving of green vegetables and the salad or two servings of salad.

QUOTE   "A man should never be ashamed to own he had been in the wrong, which is to say, in other words, that he is wiser today than he was yesterday." — *Alexander Pope*

GOAL FOR THE WEEK:

STATISTICS	weight	waist"	hips"
Beginning:	_____	_____	_____
End:	_____	_____	_____

199

JULY 8	BREAKFAST	LUNCH	DINNER	SNACKS
S M T W T F S Carbohydrate Total per Meal: B _____ L _____ D _____ S _____ Daily Carbohydrate Total: _____				
	Fluids: oz.	Fluids: oz.	Fluids: oz.	Fluids: oz.
	Vit / Min / Supp:			

JULY 9	BREAKFAST	LUNCH	DINNER	SNACKS
S M T W T F S Carbohydrate Total per Meal: B _____ L _____ D _____ S _____ Daily Carbohydrate Total: _____				
	Fluids: oz.	Fluids: oz.	Fluids: oz.	Fluids: oz.
	Vit / Min / Supp:			

JULY 10	BREAKFAST	LUNCH	DINNER	SNACKS
S M T W T F S Carbohydrate Total per Meal: B _____ L _____ D _____ S _____ Daily Carbohydrate Total: _____				
	Fluids: oz.	Fluids: oz.	Fluids: oz.	Fluids: oz.
	Vit / Min / Supp:			

JULY 11	BREAKFAST	LUNCH	DINNER	SNACKS
S M T W T F S Carbohydrate Total per Meal: B _____ L _____ D _____ S _____ Daily Carbohydrate Total: _____				
	Fluids: oz.	Fluids: oz.	Fluids: oz.	Fluids: oz.
	Vit / Min / Supp:			

EXERCISE GOALS: _____

EXERCISE DONE: _____

JULY 12	BREAKFAST	LUNCH	DINNER	SNACKS
S M T W T F S Carbohydrate Total per Meal: B _____ L _____ D _____ S _____				
Daily Carbohydrate Total: _____	Fluids: _____ oz.	Fluids: _____ oz.	Fluids: _____ oz.	Fluids: _____ oz.
	Vit / Min / Supp:			

JULY 13	BREAKFAST	LUNCH	DINNER	SNACKS
S M T W T F S Carbohydrate Total per Meal: B _____ L _____ D _____ S _____				
Daily Carbohydrate Total: _____	Fluids: _____ oz.	Fluids: _____ oz.	Fluids: _____ oz.	Fluids: _____ oz.
	Vit / Min / Supp:			

JULY 14	BREAKFAST	LUNCH	DINNER	SNACKS
S M T W T F S Carbohydrate Total per Meal: B _____ L _____ D _____ S _____				
Daily Carbohydrate Total: _____	Fluids: _____ oz.	Fluids: _____ oz.	Fluids: _____ oz.	Fluids: _____ oz.
	Vit / Min / Supp:			

TIP Carbohydrate bargains of three or fewer grams: 6 fresh asparagus spears (2.4), 1 cup chopped raw broccoli (2.2), ½ medium cucumber (3), ½ cup raw mushroom pieces (1.1), ½ cup canned asparagus (2.9), ½ cup canned bamboo shoots (2.3).

QUOTE "What we learn to do we learn by doing." — *Aristotle*

GOAL FOR THE WEEK:

STATISTICS	weight	waist"	hips"
Beginning:	_____	_____	_____
End:	_____	_____	_____

JULY 15	BREAKFAST	LUNCH	DINNER	SNACKS
S M T W T F S Carbohydrate Total per Meal: B _____ L _____ D _____ S _____				
Daily Carbohydrate Total: _____	Fluids: _____ oz.	Fluids: _____ oz.	Fluids: _____ oz.	Fluids: _____ oz.
	Vit / Min / Supp:			

JULY 16	BREAKFAST	LUNCH	DINNER	SNACKS
S M T W T F S Carbohydrate Total per Meal: B _____ L _____ D _____ S _____				
Daily Carbohydrate Total: _____	Fluids: _____ oz.	Fluids: _____ oz.	Fluids: _____ oz.	Fluids: _____ oz.
	Vit / Min / Supp:			

JULY 17	BREAKFAST	LUNCH	DINNER	SNACKS
S M T W T F S Carbohydrate Total per Meal: B _____ L _____ D _____ S _____				
Daily Carbohydrate Total: _____	Fluids: _____ oz.	Fluids: _____ oz.	Fluids: _____ oz.	Fluids: _____ oz.
	Vit / Min / Supp:			

JULY 18	BREAKFAST	LUNCH	DINNER	SNACKS
S M T W T F S Carbohydrate Total per Meal: B _____ L _____ D _____ S _____				
Daily Carbohydrate Total: _____	Fluids: _____ oz.	Fluids: _____ oz.	Fluids: _____ oz.	Fluids: _____ oz.
	Vit / Min / Supp:			

EXERCISE GOALS: _____

EXERCISE DONE: _____

202

JULY 19	BREAKFAST	LUNCH	DINNER	SNACKS
S M T W T F S Carbohydrate Total per Meal: B _____ L _____ D _____ S _____				
Daily Carbohydrate Total: _____	Fluids: ___ oz.	Fluids: ___ oz.	Fluids: ___ oz.	Fluids: ___ oz.
	Vit / Min / Supp:			

JULY 20	BREAKFAST	LUNCH	DINNER	SNACKS
S M T W T F S Carbohydrate Total per Meal: B _____ L _____ D _____ S _____				
Daily Carbohydrate Total: _____	Fluids: ___ oz.	Fluids: ___ oz.	Fluids: ___ oz.	Fluids: ___ oz.
	Vit / Min / Supp:			

JULY 21	BREAKFAST	LUNCH	DINNER	SNACKS
S M T W T F S Carbohydrate Total per Meal: B _____ L _____ D _____ S _____				
Daily Carbohydrate Total: _____	Fluids: ___ oz.	Fluids: ___ oz.	Fluids: ___ oz.	Fluids: ___ oz.
	Vit / Min / Supp:			

TIP If you have a sweet attack—wait ten minutes. If you still must have a sweet, eat ¼ cup cottage cheese or a few cubes of cheddar cheese. It that doesn't stop it, then indulge in: 8 chocolate-covered espresso beans (5 carbohydrates), or 1 Hershey's Nugget with almonds (5), or 1 Milky Way Miniature (6).

QUOTE "Keep adding little by little and you will soon have a big hoard." — *Latin proverb*

GOAL FOR THE WEEK:

STATISTICS	weight	waist"	hips"
Beginning:	_____	_____	_____
End:	_____	_____	_____

JULY 22	BREAKFAST	LUNCH	DINNER	SNACKS
S M T W T F S Carbohydrate Total per Meal: B _____ L _____ D _____ S _____ Daily Carbohydrate Total: _____				
	Fluids: ____ oz.	Fluids: ____ oz.	Fluids: ____ oz.	Fluids: ____ oz.
	Vit / Min / Supp:			

JULY 23	BREAKFAST	LUNCH	DINNER	SNACKS
S M T W T F S Carbohydrate Total per Meal: B _____ L _____ D _____ S _____ Daily Carbohydrate Total: _____				
	Fluids: ____ oz.	Fluids: ____ oz.	Fluids: ____ oz.	Fluids: ____ oz.
	Vit / Min / Supp:			

JULY 24	BREAKFAST	LUNCH	DINNER	SNACKS
S M T W T F S Carbohydrate Total per Meal: B _____ L _____ D _____ S _____ Daily Carbohydrate Total: _____				
	Fluids: ____ oz.	Fluids: ____ oz.	Fluids: ____ oz.	Fluids: ____ oz.
	Vit / Min / Supp:			

JULY 25	BREAKFAST	LUNCH	DINNER	SNACKS
S M T W T F S Carbohydrate Total per Meal: B _____ L _____ D _____ S _____ Daily Carbohydrate Total: _____				
	Fluids: ____ oz.	Fluids: ____ oz.	Fluids: ____ oz.	Fluids: ____ oz.
	Vit / Min / Supp:			

EXERCISE GOALS: _____

EXERCISE DONE: _____

JULY 26	BREAKFAST	LUNCH	DINNER	SNACKS
S M T W T F S Carbohydrate Total per Meal: B _____ L _____ D _____ S _____ Daily Carbohydrate Total: _____				
	Fluids: oz.	Fluids: oz.	Fluids: oz.	Fluids: oz.
	Vit / Min / Supp:			

JULY 27	BREAKFAST	LUNCH	DINNER	SNACKS
S M T W T F S Carbohydrate Total per Meal: B _____ L _____ D _____ S _____ Daily Carbohydrate Total: _____				
	Fluids: oz.	Fluids: oz.	Fluids: oz.	Fluids: oz.
	Vit / Min / Supp:			

JULY 28	BREAKFAST	LUNCH	DINNER	SNACKS
S M T W T F S Carbohydrate Total per Meal: B _____ L _____ D _____ S _____ Daily Carbohydrate Total: _____				
	Fluids: oz.	Fluids: oz.	Fluids: oz.	Fluids: oz.
	Vit / Min / Supp:			

TIP   Craving a crunch? Try unlimited pork rinds (0 carbohydrates), 5 Wheat Thins (5), ¼ cup tamari almonds (3).

QUOTE   "My imperfections and failures are as much a blessing from God as my successes and my talents, I lay them both at his feet." — *Mahatma Gandhi*

GOAL FOR THE WEEK:

STATISTICS   weight   waist"   hips"
Beginning: _____   _____   _____
End: _____   _____   _____

JULY 29	BREAKFAST	LUNCH	DINNER	SNACKS
S M T W T F S Carbohydrate Total per Meal: B _____ L _____ D _____ S _____ Daily Carbohydrate Total: _____				
	Fluids: ___ oz.	Fluids: ___ oz.	Fluids: ___ oz.	Fluids: ___ oz.
	Vit / Min / Supp:			

JULY 30	BREAKFAST	LUNCH	DINNER	SNACKS
S M T W T F S Carbohydrate Total per Meal: B _____ L _____ D _____ S _____ Daily Carbohydrate Total: _____				
	Fluids: ___ oz.	Fluids: ___ oz.	Fluids: ___ oz.	Fluids: ___ oz.
	Vit / Min / Supp:			

JULY 31	BREAKFAST	LUNCH	DINNER	SNACKS
S M T W T F S Carbohydrate Total per Meal: B _____ L _____ D _____ S _____ Daily Carbohydrate Total: _____				
	Fluids: ___ oz.	Fluids: ___ oz.	Fluids: ___ oz.	Fluids: ___ oz.
	Vit / Min / Supp:			

AUGUST 1	BREAKFAST	LUNCH	DINNER	SNACKS
S M T W T F S Carbohydrate Total per Meal: B _____ L _____ D _____ S _____ Daily Carbohydrate Total: _____				
	Fluids: ___ oz.	Fluids: ___ oz.	Fluids: ___ oz.	Fluids: ___ oz.
	Vit / Min / Supp:			

EXERCISE GOALS: _____

EXERCISE DONE: _____

AUGUST 2	BREAKFAST	LUNCH	DINNER	SNACKS
S M T W T F S Carbohydrate Total per Meal: B _____ L _____ D _____ S _____ Daily Carbohydrate Total: _____				
	Fluids: oz.	Fluids: oz.	Fluids: oz.	Fluids: oz.
	Vit / Min / Supp:			

AUGUST 3	BREAKFAST	LUNCH	DINNER	SNACKS
S M T W T F S Carbohydrate Total per Meal: B _____ L _____ D _____ S _____ Daily Carbohydrate Total: _____				
	Fluids: oz.	Fluids: oz.	Fluids: oz.	Fluids: oz.
	Vit / Min / Supp:			

AUGUST 4	BREAKFAST	LUNCH	DINNER	SNACKS
S M T W T F S Carbohydrate Total per Meal: B _____ L _____ D _____ S _____ Daily Carbohydrate Total: _____				
	Fluids: oz.	Fluids: oz.	Fluids: oz.	Fluids: oz.
	Vit / Min / Supp:			

TIP   Visualize clearly and vividly the changes you wish to take place. You will set in motion all kinds of sub-conscious activity that will work behind the scenes to make your visual pictures a reality.

QUOTE   "Let one therefore keep the mind pure, for what a man thinks, that he becomes." — *The Upanishads*

GOAL FOR THE WEEK:

STATISTICS	weight	waist"	hips"
Beginning:	_____	_____	_____
End:	_____	_____	_____

AUGUST 5	BREAKFAST	LUNCH	DINNER	SNACKS
S M T W T F S Carbohydrate Total per Meal: B _____ L _____ D _____ S _____ Daily Carbohydrate Total: _____				
	Fluids: oz.	Fluids: oz.	Fluids: oz.	Fluids: oz.
	Vit / Min / Supp:			

AUGUST 6	BREAKFAST	LUNCH	DINNER	SNACKS
S M T W T F S Carbohydrate Total per Meal: B _____ L _____ D _____ S _____ Daily Carbohydrate Total: _____				
	Fluids: oz.	Fluids: oz.	Fluids: oz.	Fluids: oz.
	Vit / Min / Supp:			

AUGUST 7	BREAKFAST	LUNCH	DINNER	SNACKS
S M T W T F S Carbohydrate Total per Meal: B _____ L _____ D _____ S _____ Daily Carbohydrate Total: _____				
	Fluids: oz.	Fluids: oz.	Fluids: oz.	Fluids: oz.
	Vit / Min / Supp:			

AUGUST 8	BREAKFAST	LUNCH	DINNER	SNACKS
S M T W T F S Carbohydrate Total per Meal: B _____ L _____ D _____ S _____ Daily Carbohydrate Total: _____				
	Fluids: oz.	Fluids: oz.	Fluids: oz.	Fluids: oz.
	Vit / Min / Supp:			

EXERCISE GOALS: _____

EXERCISE DONE: _____

AUGUST 9	BREAKFAST	LUNCH	DINNER	SNACKS
S M T W T F S Carbohydrate Total per Meal: B _____ L _____ D _____ S _____ Daily Carbohydrate Total: _____				
	Fluids: oz.	Fluids: oz.	Fluids: oz.	Fluids: oz.
	Vit / Min / Supp:			

AUGUST 10	BREAKFAST	LUNCH	DINNER	SNACKS
S M T W T F S Carbohydrate Total per Meal: B _____ L _____ D _____ S _____ Daily Carbohydrate Total: _____				
	Fluids: oz.	Fluids: oz.	Fluids: oz.	Fluids: oz.
	Vit / Min / Supp:			

AUGUST 11	BREAKFAST	LUNCH	DINNER	SNACKS
S M T W T F S Carbohydrate Total per Meal: B _____ L _____ D _____ S _____ Daily Carbohydrate Total: _____				
	Fluids: oz.	Fluids: oz.	Fluids: oz.	Fluids: oz.
	Vit / Min / Supp:			

TIP   Make the commitment that if it goes into your mouth, it goes into your journal. Studies have shown that people who commit to keeping an honest and accurate diary of nutrition and exercise are as much as four times more successful than people who will not.

QUOTE   "We are what we repeatedly do. Excellence, then, is not an act, but a habit." — *Aristotle*

GOAL FOR THE WEEK:

STATISTICS	weight	waist"	hips"
Beginning:	_____	_____	_____
End:	_____	_____	_____

AUGUST 12	BREAKFAST	LUNCH	DINNER	SNACKS
S M T W T F S Carbohydrate Total per Meal: B _____ L _____ D _____ S _____ Daily Carbohydrate Total: _____				
	Fluids: oz.	Fluids: oz.	Fluids: oz.	Fluids: oz.
	Vit / Min / Supp:			

AUGUST 13	BREAKFAST	LUNCH	DINNER	SNACKS
S M T W T F S Carbohydrate Total per Meal: B _____ L _____ D _____ S _____ Daily Carbohydrate Total: _____				
	Fluids: oz.	Fluids: oz.	Fluids: oz.	Fluids: oz.
	Vit / Min / Supp:			

AUGUST 14	BREAKFAST	LUNCH	DINNER	SNACKS
S M T W T F S Carbohydrate Total per Meal: B _____ L _____ D _____ S _____ Daily Carbohydrate Total: _____				
	Fluids: oz.	Fluids: oz.	Fluids: oz.	Fluids: oz.
	Vit / Min / Supp:			

AUGUST 15	BREAKFAST	LUNCH	DINNER	SNACKS
S M T W T F S Carbohydrate Total per Meal: B _____ L _____ D _____ S _____ Daily Carbohydrate Total: _____				
	Fluids: oz.	Fluids: oz.	Fluids: oz.	Fluids: oz.
	Vit / Min / Supp:			

EXERCISE GOALS: _____

EXERCISE DONE: _____

AUGUST 16	BREAKFAST	LUNCH	DINNER	SNACKS
S M T W T F S Carbohydrate Total per Meal: B _____ L _____ D _____ S _____				
Daily Carbohydrate Total: _____	Fluids: oz.	Fluids: oz.	Fluids: oz.	Fluids: oz.
	Vit / Min / Supp:			

AUGUST 17	BREAKFAST	LUNCH	DINNER	SNACKS
S M T W T F S Carbohydrate Total per Meal: B _____ L _____ D _____ S _____				
Daily Carbohydrate Total: _____	Fluids: oz.	Fluids: oz.	Fluids: oz.	Fluids: oz.
	Vit / Min / Supp:			

AUGUST 18	BREAKFAST	LUNCH	DINNER	SNACKS
S M T W T F S Carbohydrate Total per Meal: B _____ L _____ D _____ S _____				
Daily Carbohydrate Total: _____	Fluids: oz.	Fluids: oz.	Fluids: oz.	Fluids: oz.
	Vit / Min / Supp:			

TIP   If you snack, remember to count those carbohydrates in your daily total. A gram here and a gram there can add up quickly.

QUOTE   "Do what you can, with what you have, where you are." — *Theodore Roosevelt*

GOAL FOR THE WEEK:

STATISTICS	weight	waist"	hips"
Beginning:	_____	_____	_____
End:	_____	_____	_____

AUGUST 19	BREAKFAST	LUNCH	DINNER	SNACKS
S M T W T F S Carbohydrate Total per Meal: B _____ L _____ D _____ S _____ Daily Carbohydrate Total: _____				
	Fluids: ____ oz.	Fluids: ____ oz.	Fluids: ____ oz.	Fluids: ____ oz.
	Vit / Min / Supp:			

AUGUST 20	BREAKFAST	LUNCH	DINNER	SNACKS
S M T W T F S Carbohydrate Total per Meal: B _____ L _____ D _____ S _____ Daily Carbohydrate Total: _____				
	Fluids: ____ oz.	Fluids: ____ oz.	Fluids: ____ oz.	Fluids: ____ oz.
	Vit / Min / Supp:			

AUGUST 21	BREAKFAST	LUNCH	DINNER	SNACKS
S M T W T F S Carbohydrate Total per Meal: B _____ L _____ D _____ S _____ Daily Carbohydrate Total: _____				
	Fluids: ____ oz.	Fluids: ____ oz.	Fluids: ____ oz.	Fluids: ____ oz.
	Vit / Min / Supp:			

AUGUST 22	BREAKFAST	LUNCH	DINNER	SNACKS
S M T W T F S Carbohydrate Total per Meal: B _____ L _____ D _____ S _____ Daily Carbohydrate Total: _____				
	Fluids: ____ oz.	Fluids: ____ oz.	Fluids: ____ oz.	Fluids: ____ oz.
	Vit / Min / Supp:			

EXERCISE GOALS: _____

EXERCISE DONE: _____

AUGUST 23	BREAKFAST	LUNCH	DINNER	SNACKS
S M T W T F S Carbohydrate Total per Meal: B _____ L _____ D _____ S _____				
Daily Carbohydrate Total: _____	Fluids: oz.	Fluids: oz.	Fluids: oz.	Fluids: oz.
	Vit / Min / Supp:			

AUGUST 24	BREAKFAST	LUNCH	DINNER	SNACKS
S M T W T F S Carbohydrate Total per Meal: B _____ L _____ D _____ S _____				
Daily Carbohydrate Total: _____	Fluids: oz.	Fluids: oz.	Fluids: oz.	Fluids: oz.
	Vit / Min / Supp:			

AUGUST 25	BREAKFAST	LUNCH	DINNER	SNACKS
S M T W T F S Carbohydrate Total per Meal: B _____ L _____ D _____ S _____				
Daily Carbohydrate Total: _____	Fluids: oz.	Fluids: oz.	Fluids: oz.	Fluids: oz.
	Vit / Min / Supp:			

TIP   Entertaining friends or business associates for drinks? Serve a chunk of cheese, pickled asparagus and/or green beans, several kinds of olives, and some deviled egg halves, and you're still on the low-carb wagon—unless, of course, you eat more than your share!

QUOTE   "This above all: to thine own self be true." — *William Shakespeare*

GOAL FOR THE WEEK:

STATISTICS   weight   waist"   hips"
Beginning: _____   _____   _____
End: _____   _____   _____

AUGUST 26	BREAKFAST	LUNCH	DINNER	SNACKS
S M T W T F S Carbohydrate Total per Meal: B _____ L _____ D _____ S _____ Daily Carbohydrate Total: _____				
	Fluids: oz.	Fluids: oz.	Fluids: oz.	Fluids: oz.
	Vit / Min / Supp:			

AUGUST 27	BREAKFAST	LUNCH	DINNER	SNACKS
S M T W T F S Carbohydrate Total per Meal: B _____ L _____ D _____ S _____ Daily Carbohydrate Total: _____				
	Fluids: oz.	Fluids: oz.	Fluids: oz.	Fluids: oz.
	Vit / Min / Supp:			

AUGUST 28	BREAKFAST	LUNCH	DINNER	SNACKS
S M T W T F S Carbohydrate Total per Meal: B _____ L _____ D _____ S _____ Daily Carbohydrate Total: _____				
	Fluids: oz.	Fluids: oz.	Fluids: oz.	Fluids: oz.
	Vit / Min / Supp:			

AUGUST 29	BREAKFAST	LUNCH	DINNER	SNACKS
S M T W T F S Carbohydrate Total per Meal: B _____ L _____ D _____ S _____ Daily Carbohydrate Total: _____				
	Fluids: oz.	Fluids: oz.	Fluids: oz.	Fluids: oz.
	Vit / Min / Supp:			

EXERCISE GOALS: _____

EXERCISE DONE: _____

AUGUST 30	BREAKFAST	LUNCH	DINNER	SNACKS
S M T W T F S Carbohydrate Total per Meal: B _____ L _____ D _____ S _____				
Daily Carbohydrate Total: _____	Fluids: ____ oz.	Fluids: ____ oz.	Fluids: ____ oz.	Fluids: ____ oz.
	Vit / Min / Supp:			

AUGUST 31	BREAKFAST	LUNCH	DINNER	SNACKS
S M T W T F S Carbohydrate Total per Meal: B _____ L _____ D _____ S _____				
Daily Carbohydrate Total: _____	Fluids: ____ oz.	Fluids: ____ oz.	Fluids: ____ oz.	Fluids: ____ oz.
	Vit / Min / Supp:			

SEPTEMBER 1	BREAKFAST	LUNCH	DINNER	SNACKS
S M T W T F S Carbohydrate Total per Meal: B _____ L _____ D _____ S _____				
Daily Carbohydrate Total: _____	Fluids: ____ oz.	Fluids: ____ oz.	Fluids: ____ oz.	Fluids: ____ oz.
	Vit / Min / Supp:			

TIP   There are more carbohydrates in nondairy creamers than in either cream or half-and-half. If you wish, lighten your tea or coffee with cream or half-and-half.

QUOTE   "Our doubts are traitors, and make us lose the good we oft might win by fearing to attempt." — *William Shakespeare*

GOAL FOR THE WEEK:

STATISTICS   weight   waist"   hips"
Beginning: _____   _____   _____
End: _____   _____   _____

SEPTEMBER 2	BREAKFAST	LUNCH	DINNER	SNACKS
S M T W T F S Carbohydrate Total per Meal: B _____ L _____ D _____ S _____ Daily Carbohydrate Total: _____				
	Fluids: oz.	Fluids: oz.	Fluids: oz.	Fluids: oz.
	Vit / Min / Supp:			

SEPTEMBER 3	BREAKFAST	LUNCH	DINNER	SNACKS
S M T W T F S Carbohydrate Total per Meal: B _____ L _____ D _____ S _____ Daily Carbohydrate Total: _____				
	Fluids: oz.	Fluids: oz.	Fluids: oz.	Fluids: oz.
	Vit / Min / Supp:			

SEPTEMBER 4	BREAKFAST	LUNCH	DINNER	SNACKS
S M T W T F S Carbohydrate Total per Meal: B _____ L _____ D _____ S _____ Daily Carbohydrate Total: _____				
	Fluids: oz.	Fluids: oz.	Fluids: oz.	Fluids: oz.
	Vit / Min / Supp:			

SEPTEMBER 5	BREAKFAST	LUNCH	DINNER	SNACKS
S M T W T F S Carbohydrate Total per Meal: B _____ L _____ D _____ S _____ Daily Carbohydrate Total: _____				
	Fluids: oz.	Fluids: oz.	Fluids: oz.	Fluids: oz.
	Vit / Min / Supp:			

EXERCISE GOALS: _____

EXERCISE DONE: _____

SEPTEMBER 6	BREAKFAST	LUNCH	DINNER	SNACKS
S M T W T F S Carbohydrate Total per Meal: B _____ L _____ D _____ S _____				
Daily Carbohydrate Total: _____	Fluids: oz.	Fluids: oz.	Fluids: oz.	Fluids: oz.
	Vit / Min / Supp:			

SEPTEMBER 7	BREAKFAST	LUNCH	DINNER	SNACKS
S M T W T F S Carbohydrate Total per Meal: B _____ L _____ D _____ S _____				
Daily Carbohydrate Total: _____	Fluids: oz.	Fluids: oz.	Fluids: oz.	Fluids: oz.
	Vit / Min / Supp:			

SEPTEMBER 8	BREAKFAST	LUNCH	DINNER	SNACKS
S M T W T F S Carbohydrate Total per Meal: B _____ L _____ D _____ S _____				
Daily Carbohydrate Total: _____	Fluids: oz.	Fluids: oz.	Fluids: oz.	Fluids: oz.
	Vit / Min / Supp:			

TIP   Nutritional maintenance of your health requires vigilance and effort most of the time, interspersed with occasional brief vacations from the straight and narrow.

QUOTE   "Confidence imparts a wonderful inspiration to its possessor." — *John Milton*

GOAL FOR THE WEEK:

STATISTICS	weight	waist"	hips"
Beginning:	_____	_____	_____
End:	_____	_____	_____

SEPTEMBER 9	BREAKFAST	LUNCH	DINNER	SNACKS
S M T W T F S Carbohydrate Total per Meal: B _____ L _____ D _____ S _____				
Daily Carbohydrate	Fluids: oz.	Fluids: oz.	Fluids: oz.	Fluids: oz.
Total: _____	Vit / Min / Supp:			

SEPTEMBER 10	BREAKFAST	LUNCH	DINNER	SNACKS
S M T W T F S Carbohydrate Total per Meal: B _____ L _____ D _____ S _____				
Daily Carbohydrate	Fluids: oz.	Fluids: oz.	Fluids: oz.	Fluids: oz.
Total: _____	Vit / Min / Supp:			

SEPTEMBER 11	BREAKFAST	LUNCH	DINNER	SNACKS
S M T W T F S Carbohydrate Total per Meal: B _____ L _____ D _____ S _____				
Daily Carbohydrate	Fluids: oz.	Fluids: oz.	Fluids: oz.	Fluids: oz.
Total: _____	Vit / Min / Supp:			

SEPTEMBER 12	BREAKFAST	LUNCH	DINNER	SNACKS
S M T W T F S Carbohydrate Total per Meal: B _____ L _____ D _____ S _____				
Daily Carbohydrate	Fluids: oz.	Fluids: oz.	Fluids: oz.	Fluids: oz.
Total: _____	Vit / Min / Supp:			

EXERCISE GOALS: _____

EXERCISE DONE: _____

SEPTEMBER 13	BREAKFAST	LUNCH	DINNER	SNACKS
S M T W T F S Carbohydrate Total per Meal: B _____ L _____ D _____ S _____ Daily Carbohydrate Total: _____				
	Fluids: _____ oz.	Fluids: _____ oz.	Fluids: _____ oz.	Fluids: _____ oz.
	Vit / Min / Supp:			

SEPTEMBER 14	BREAKFAST	LUNCH	DINNER	SNACKS
S M T W T F S Carbohydrate Total per Meal: B _____ L _____ D _____ S _____ Daily Carbohydrate Total: _____				
	Fluids: _____ oz.	Fluids: _____ oz.	Fluids: _____ oz.	Fluids: _____ oz.
	Vit / Min / Supp:			

SEPTEMBER 15	BREAKFAST	LUNCH	DINNER	SNACKS
S M T W T F S Carbohydrate Total per Meal: B _____ L _____ D _____ S _____ Daily Carbohydrate Total: _____				
	Fluids: _____ oz.	Fluids: _____ oz.	Fluids: _____ oz.	Fluids: _____ oz.
	Vit / Min / Supp:			

TIP   Plan your diet vacations. Select several times a year to celebrate by fully partaking. Whether it's your birthday, Christmas, a romantic getaway, or a wedding, plan for it, recover from it, and return to maintenance. Knowing that you have a planned vacation from maintenance somehow makes the day-by-day sacrifices less burdensome.

QUOTE   "True hope is based on energy of character. A strong mind always hopes." — *Karl von Knebel*

GOAL FOR THE WEEK:

STATISTICS	weight	waist"	hips"
Beginning:	_____	_____	_____
End:	_____	_____	_____

SEPTEMBER 16	BREAKFAST	LUNCH	DINNER	SNACKS
S M T W T F S Carbohydrate Total per Meal: B _____ L _____ D _____ S _____				
Daily Carbohydrate	Fluids: oz.	Fluids: oz.	Fluids: oz.	Fluids: oz.
Total: _____	Vit / Min / Supp:			

SEPTEMBER 17	BREAKFAST	LUNCH	DINNER	SNACKS
S M T W T F S Carbohydrate Total per Meal: B _____ L _____ D _____ S _____				
Daily Carbohydrate	Fluids: oz.	Fluids: oz.	Fluids: oz.	Fluids: oz.
Total: _____	Vit / Min / Supp:			

SEPTEMBER 18	BREAKFAST	LUNCH	DINNER	SNACKS
S M T W T F S Carbohydrate Total per Meal: B _____ L _____ D _____ S _____				
Daily Carbohydrate	Fluids: oz.	Fluids: oz.	Fluids: oz.	Fluids: oz.
Total: _____	Vit / Min / Supp:			

SEPTEMBER 19	BREAKFAST	LUNCH	DINNER	SNACKS
S M T W T F S Carbohydrate Total per Meal: B _____ L _____ D _____ S _____				
Daily Carbohydrate	Fluids: oz.	Fluids: oz.	Fluids: oz.	Fluids: oz.
Total: _____	Vit / Min / Supp:			

EXERCISE GOALS: _____

EXERCISE DONE: _____

SEPTEMBER 20	BREAKFAST	LUNCH	DINNER	SNACKS
S M T W T F S Carbohydrate Total per Meal: B _____ L _____ D _____ S _____				
Daily Carbohydrate Total: _____	Fluids: ____ oz.	Fluids: ____ oz.	Fluids: ____ oz.	Fluids: ____ oz.
	Vit / Min / Supp:			

SEPTEMBER 21	BREAKFAST	LUNCH	DINNER	SNACKS
S M T W T F S Carbohydrate Total per Meal: B _____ L _____ D _____ S _____				
Daily Carbohydrate Total: _____	Fluids: ____ oz.	Fluids: ____ oz.	Fluids: ____ oz.	Fluids: ____ oz.
	Vit / Min / Supp:			

SEPTEMBER 22	BREAKFAST	LUNCH	DINNER	SNACKS
S M T W T F S Carbohydrate Total per Meal: B _____ L _____ D _____ S _____				
Daily Carbohydrate Total: _____	Fluids: ____ oz.	Fluids: ____ oz.	Fluids: ____ oz.	Fluids: ____ oz.
	Vit / Min / Supp:			

TIP   Six pounds of fat takes up almost a gallon of space in volume!

QUOTE   "I steer my bark with hope ahead and fear astern." — *Thomas Jefferson*

GOAL FOR THE WEEK:

STATISTICS	weight	waist"	hips"
Beginning:	_____	_____	_____
End:	_____	_____	_____

SEPTEMBER 23	BREAKFAST	LUNCH	DINNER	SNACKS
S M T W T F S Carbohydrate Total per Meal: B _____ L _____ D _____ S _____				
Daily Carbohydrate Total: _____	Fluids: oz.	Fluids: oz.	Fluids: oz.	Fluids: oz.
	Vit / Min / Supp:			

SEPTEMBER 24	BREAKFAST	LUNCH	DINNER	SNACKS
S M T W T F S Carbohydrate Total per Meal: B _____ L _____ D _____ S _____				
Daily Carbohydrate Total: _____	Fluids: oz.	Fluids: oz.	Fluids: oz.	Fluids: oz.
	Vit / Min / Supp:			

SEPTEMBER 25	BREAKFAST	LUNCH	DINNER	SNACKS
S M T W T F S Carbohydrate Total per Meal: B _____ L _____ D _____ S _____				
Daily Carbohydrate Total: _____	Fluids: oz.	Fluids: oz.	Fluids: oz.	Fluids: oz.
	Vit / Min / Supp:			

SEPTEMBER 26	BREAKFAST	LUNCH	DINNER	SNACKS
S M T W T F S Carbohydrate Total per Meal: B _____ L _____ D _____ S _____				
Daily Carbohydrate Total: _____	Fluids: oz.	Fluids: oz.	Fluids: oz.	Fluids: oz.
	Vit / Min / Supp:			

EXERCISE GOALS: _____

EXERCISE DONE: _____

SEPTEMBER 27	BREAKFAST	LUNCH	DINNER	SNACKS
S M T W T F S Carbohydrate Total per Meal: B _____ L _____ D _____ S _____				
Daily Carbohydrate Total: _____	Fluids: _____ oz.	Fluids: _____ oz.	Fluids: _____ oz.	Fluids: _____ oz.
	Vit / Min / Supp:			

SEPTEMBER 28	BREAKFAST	LUNCH	DINNER	SNACKS
S M T W T F S Carbohydrate Total per Meal: B _____ L _____ D _____ S _____				
Daily Carbohydrate Total: _____	Fluids: _____ oz.	Fluids: _____ oz.	Fluids: _____ oz.	Fluids: _____ oz.
	Vit / Min / Supp:			

SEPTEMBER 29	BREAKFAST	LUNCH	DINNER	SNACKS
S M T W T F S Carbohydrate Total per Meal: B _____ L _____ D _____ S _____				
Daily Carbohydrate Total: _____	Fluids: _____ oz.	Fluids: _____ oz.	Fluids: _____ oz.	Fluids: _____ oz.
	Vit / Min / Supp:			

TIP   Which would you rather have for under 7 grams? 7 Skittles = 1 marshmallow = $\frac{1}{2}$ Reese's peanut butter cup = $\frac{1}{2}$ cup fresh berries = $\frac{1}{2}$ cup grapes = 14 cups fresh lettuce = 3 cups raw broccoli.

QUOTE   "The natural flights of the human mind are not from pleasure to pleasure, but from hope to hope."
— Samuel Johnson

GOAL FOR THE WEEK:

STATISTICS	weight	waist"	hips"
Beginning:	_____	_____	_____
End:	_____	_____	_____

SEPTEMBER 30	BREAKFAST	LUNCH	DINNER	SNACKS
S M T W T F S Carbohydrate Total per Meal: B _____ L _____ D _____ S _____ Daily Carbohydrate Total: _____				
	Fluids: ____ oz.	Fluids: ____ oz.	Fluids: ____ oz.	Fluids: ____ oz.
	Vit / Min / Supp:			

OCTOBER 1	BREAKFAST	LUNCH	DINNER	SNACKS
S M T W T F S Carbohydrate Total per Meal: B _____ L _____ D _____ S _____ Daily Carbohydrate Total: _____				
	Fluids: ____ oz.	Fluids: ____ oz.	Fluids: ____ oz.	Fluids: ____ oz.
	Vit / Min / Supp:			

OCTOBER 2	BREAKFAST	LUNCH	DINNER	SNACKS
S M T W T F S Carbohydrate Total per Meal: B _____ L _____ D _____ S _____ Daily Carbohydrate Total: _____				
	Fluids: ____ oz.	Fluids: ____ oz.	Fluids: ____ oz.	Fluids: ____ oz.
	Vit / Min / Supp:			

OCTOBER 3	BREAKFAST	LUNCH	DINNER	SNACKS
S M T W T F S Carbohydrate Total per Meal: B _____ L _____ D _____ S _____ Daily Carbohydrate Total: _____				
	Fluids: ____ oz.	Fluids: ____ oz.	Fluids: ____ oz.	Fluids: ____ oz.
	Vit / Min / Supp:			

EXERCISE GOALS: _____

EXERCISE DONE: _____

OCTOBER 4	BREAKFAST	LUNCH	DINNER	SNACKS
S M T W T F S Carbohydrate Total per Meal: B _____ L _____ D _____ S _____				
Daily Carbohydrate Total: _____	Fluids: _____ oz.	Fluids: _____ oz.	Fluids: _____ oz.	Fluids: _____ oz.
	Vit / Min / Supp:			

OCTOBER 5	BREAKFAST	LUNCH	DINNER	SNACKS
S M T W T F S Carbohydrate Total per Meal: B _____ L _____ D _____ S _____				
Daily Carbohydrate Total: _____	Fluids: _____ oz.	Fluids: _____ oz.	Fluids: _____ oz.	Fluids: _____ oz.
	Vit / Min / Supp:			

OCTOBER 6	BREAKFAST	LUNCH	DINNER	SNACKS
S M T W T F S Carbohydrate Total per Meal: B _____ L _____ D _____ S _____				
Daily Carbohydrate Total: _____	Fluids: _____ oz.	Fluids: _____ oz.	Fluids: _____ oz.	Fluids: _____ oz.
	Vit / Min / Supp:			

TIP   You may drink your coffee, tea, or diet cola caffeinated or decaffeinated unless you are caffeine sensitive.

QUOTE   "Hope is itself a species of happiness, and, perhaps, the chief happiness which this world affords."
— Samuel Johnson

GOAL FOR THE WEEK:

STATISTICS	weight	waist"	hips"
Beginning:	_____	_____	_____
End:	_____	_____	_____

OCTOBER 7	BREAKFAST	LUNCH	DINNER	SNACKS
S M T W T F S Carbohydrate Total per Meal: B _____ L _____ D _____ S _____ Daily Carbohydrate Total: _____				
	Fluids: oz.	Fluids: oz.	Fluids: oz.	Fluids: oz.
	Vit / Min / Supp:			

OCTOBER 8	BREAKFAST	LUNCH	DINNER	SNACKS
S M T W T F S Carbohydrate Total per Meal: B _____ L _____ D _____ S _____ Daily Carbohydrate Total: _____				
	Fluids: oz.	Fluids: oz.	Fluids: oz.	Fluids: oz.
	Vit / Min / Supp:			

OCTOBER 9	BREAKFAST	LUNCH	DINNER	SNACKS
S M T W T F S Carbohydrate Total per Meal: B _____ L _____ D _____ S _____ Daily Carbohydrate Total: _____				
	Fluids: oz.	Fluids: oz.	Fluids: oz.	Fluids: oz.
	Vit / Min / Supp:			

OCTOBER 10	BREAKFAST	LUNCH	DINNER	SNACKS
S M T W T F S Carbohydrate Total per Meal: B _____ L _____ D _____ S _____ Daily Carbohydrate Total: _____				
	Fluids: oz.	Fluids: oz.	Fluids: oz.	Fluids: oz.
	Vit / Min / Supp:			

EXERCISE GOALS: _____

EXERCISE DONE: _____

OCTOBER 11	BREAKFAST	LUNCH	DINNER	SNACKS
S M T W T F S Carbohydrate Total per Meal: B _____ L _____ D _____ S _____				
Daily Carbohydrate Total: _____	Fluids: _____ oz.	Fluids: _____ oz.	Fluids: _____ oz.	Fluids: _____ oz.
	Vit / Min / Supp:			

OCTOBER 12	BREAKFAST	LUNCH	DINNER	SNACKS
S M T W T F S Carbohydrate Total per Meal: B _____ L _____ D _____ S _____				
Daily Carbohydrate Total: _____	Fluids: _____ oz.	Fluids: _____ oz.	Fluids: _____ oz.	Fluids: _____ oz.
	Vit / Min / Supp:			

OCTOBER 13	BREAKFAST	LUNCH	DINNER	SNACKS
S M T W T F S Carbohydrate Total per Meal: B _____ L _____ D _____ S _____				
Daily Carbohydrate Total: _____	Fluids: _____ oz.	Fluids: _____ oz.	Fluids: _____ oz.	Fluids: _____ oz.
	Vit / Min / Supp:			

TIP   The amount of fat on the body of an average person weighing 150 pounds contains enough energy to allow that person to walk from Miami to New York City without eating.

QUOTE   "The greatest architect and most needed is hope." — *Henry Ward Beecher*

GOAL FOR THE WEEK:

STATISTICS	weight	waist"	hips"
Beginning:	_____	_____	_____
End:	_____	_____	_____

OCTOBER 14	BREAKFAST	LUNCH	DINNER	SNACKS
S M T W T F S Carbohydrate Total per Meal: B _____ L _____ D _____ S _____				
Daily Carbohydrate	Fluids: oz.	Fluids: oz.	Fluids: oz.	Fluids: oz.
Total: _____	Vit / Min / Supp:			

OCTOBER 15	BREAKFAST	LUNCH	DINNER	SNACKS
S M T W T F S Carbohydrate Total per Meal: B _____ L _____ D _____ S _____				
Daily Carbohydrate	Fluids: oz.	Fluids: oz.	Fluids: oz.	Fluids: oz.
Total: _____	Vit / Min / Supp:			

OCTOBER 16	BREAKFAST	LUNCH	DINNER	SNACKS
S M T W T F S Carbohydrate Total per Meal: B _____ L _____ D _____ S _____				
Daily Carbohydrate	Fluids: oz.	Fluids: oz.	Fluids: oz.	Fluids: oz.
Total: _____	Vit / Min / Supp:			

OCTOBER 17	BREAKFAST	LUNCH	DINNER	SNACKS
S M T W T F S Carbohydrate Total per Meal: B _____ L _____ D _____ S _____				
Daily Carbohydrate	Fluids: oz.	Fluids: oz.	Fluids: oz.	Fluids: oz.
Total: _____	Vit / Min / Supp:			

EXERCISE GOALS: _____

EXERCISE DONE: _____

OCTOBER 18	BREAKFAST	LUNCH	DINNER	SNACKS
S M T W T F S Carbohydrate Total per Meal: B _____ L _____ D _____ S _____				
Daily Carbohydrate Total: _____	Fluids: ____ oz.	Fluids: ____ oz.	Fluids: ____ oz.	Fluids: ____ oz.
	Vit / Min / Supp:			

OCTOBER 19	BREAKFAST	LUNCH	DINNER	SNACKS
S M T W T F S Carbohydrate Total per Meal: B _____ L _____ D _____ S _____				
Daily Carbohydrate Total: _____	Fluids: ____ oz.	Fluids: ____ oz.	Fluids: ____ oz.	Fluids: ____ oz.
	Vit / Min / Supp:			

OCTOBER 20	BREAKFAST	LUNCH	DINNER	SNACKS
S M T W T F S Carbohydrate Total per Meal: B _____ L _____ D _____ S _____				
Daily Carbohydrate Total: _____	Fluids: ____ oz.	Fluids: ____ oz.	Fluids: ____ oz.	Fluids: ____ oz.
	Vit / Min / Supp:			

TIP   Create a personal mantra to tide you over during times of temptation. Repeating "Yes I can. Yes I will. This is really no big deal," or something that suits your mind-set will assist you in bringing your focus back to your success.

QUOTE   "It is worth a thousand pounds a year to have the habit of looking on the bright side of things."
— Samuel Johnson

GOAL FOR THE WEEK:

STATISTICS	weight	waist"	hips"
Beginning:	_____	_____	_____
End:	_____	_____	_____

OCTOBER 21	BREAKFAST	LUNCH	DINNER	SNACKS
S M T W T F S Carbohydrate Total per Meal: B _____ L _____ D _____ S _____ Daily Carbohydrate Total: _____				
	Fluids: _____ oz.	Fluids: _____ oz.	Fluids: _____ oz.	Fluids: _____ oz.
	Vit / Min / Supp:			

OCTOBER 22	BREAKFAST	LUNCH	DINNER	SNACKS
S M T W T F S Carbohydrate Total per Meal: B _____ L _____ D _____ S _____ Daily Carbohydrate Total: _____				
	Fluids: _____ oz.	Fluids: _____ oz.	Fluids: _____ oz.	Fluids: _____ oz.
	Vit / Min / Supp:			

OCTOBER 23	BREAKFAST	LUNCH	DINNER	SNACKS
S M T W T F S Carbohydrate Total per Meal: B _____ L _____ D _____ S _____ Daily Carbohydrate Total: _____				
	Fluids: _____ oz.	Fluids: _____ oz.	Fluids: _____ oz.	Fluids: _____ oz.
	Vit / Min / Supp:			

OCTOBER 24	BREAKFAST	LUNCH	DINNER	SNACKS
S M T W T F S Carbohydrate Total per Meal: B _____ L _____ D _____ S _____ Daily Carbohydrate Total: _____				
	Fluids: _____ oz.	Fluids: _____ oz.	Fluids: _____ oz.	Fluids: _____ oz.
	Vit / Min / Supp:			

EXERCISE GOALS: _____

EXERCISE DONE: _____

OCTOBER 25	BREAKFAST	LUNCH	DINNER	SNACKS
S M T W T F S Carbohydrate Total per Meal: B _____ L _____ D _____ S _____				
Daily Carbohydrate	Fluids: oz.	Fluids: oz.	Fluids: oz.	Fluids: oz.
Total: _____	Vit / Min / Supp:			

OCTOBER 26	BREAKFAST	LUNCH	DINNER	SNACKS
S M T W T F S Carbohydrate Total per Meal: B _____ L _____ D _____ S _____				
Daily Carbohydrate	Fluids: oz.	Fluids: oz.	Fluids: oz.	Fluids: oz.
Total: _____	Vit / Min / Supp:			

OCTOBER 27	BREAKFAST	LUNCH	DINNER	SNACKS
S M T W T F S Carbohydrate Total per Meal: B _____ L _____ D _____ S _____				
Daily Carbohydrate	Fluids: oz.	Fluids: oz.	Fluids: oz.	Fluids: oz.
Total: _____	Vit / Min / Supp:			

TIP   Encourage yourself by creating signs with your desired waist measurement, weight, or clothing size and posting them in places where you will see them often. Some suggestions are: your desk, the bathroom mirror, inside the refrigerator, on the dash of your car. Remind yourself often of your goals—a sign that says only "26" is your secret.

QUOTE   "Hope is the dream of the waking man." — *Aristotle*

GOAL FOR THE WEEK:

STATISTICS	weight	waist"	hips"
Beginning:	_____	_____	_____
End:	_____	_____	_____

OCTOBER 28	BREAKFAST	LUNCH	DINNER	SNACKS
S M T W T F S Carbohydrate Total per Meal: B _____ L _____ D _____ S _____ Daily Carbohydrate Total: _____				
	Fluids: oz.	Fluids: oz.	Fluids: oz.	Fluids: oz.
	Vit / Min / Supp:			

OCTOBER 29	BREAKFAST	LUNCH	DINNER	SNACKS
S M T W T F S Carbohydrate Total per Meal: B _____ L _____ D _____ S _____ Daily Carbohydrate Total: _____				
	Fluids: oz.	Fluids: oz.	Fluids: oz.	Fluids: oz.
	Vit / Min / Supp:			

OCTOBER 30	BREAKFAST	LUNCH	DINNER	SNACKS
S M T W T F S Carbohydrate Total per Meal: B _____ L _____ D _____ S _____ Daily Carbohydrate Total: _____				
	Fluids: oz.	Fluids: oz.	Fluids: oz.	Fluids: oz.
	Vit / Min / Supp:			

OCTOBER 31	BREAKFAST	LUNCH	DINNER	SNACKS
S M T W T F S Carbohydrate Total per Meal: B _____ L _____ D _____ S _____ Daily Carbohydrate Total: _____				
	Fluids: oz.	Fluids: oz.	Fluids: oz.	Fluids: oz.
	Vit / Min / Supp:			

EXERCISE GOALS: _____

EXERCISE DONE: _____

NOVEMBER 1	BREAKFAST	LUNCH	DINNER	SNACKS
S M T W T F S Carbohydrate Total per Meal: B _____ L _____ D _____ S _____ Daily Carbohydrate Total: _____				
	Fluids: oz.	Fluids: oz.	Fluids: oz.	Fluids: oz.
	Vit / Min / Supp:			

NOVEMBER 2	BREAKFAST	LUNCH	DINNER	SNACKS
S M T W T F S Carbohydrate Total per Meal: B _____ L _____ D _____ S _____ Daily Carbohydrate Total: _____				
	Fluids: oz.	Fluids: oz.	Fluids: oz.	Fluids: oz.
	Vit / Min / Supp:			

NOVEMBER 3	BREAKFAST	LUNCH	DINNER	SNACKS
S M T W T F S Carbohydrate Total per Meal: B _____ L _____ D _____ S _____ Daily Carbohydrate Total: _____				
	Fluids: oz.	Fluids: oz.	Fluids: oz.	Fluids: oz.
	Vit / Min / Supp:			

TIP   Celebrate your interim goals. If your goal is to lose 2 inches this week and you achieve that goal, cele-brate. Small celebrations of interim goals build your confidence in reaching your ultimate goals. Pat yourself on the back. Give yourself positive "self-talk" when your actions support your goals.

QUOTE   "A good hope is better than a bad possession." — *Old proverb*

GOAL FOR THE WEEK:

STATISTICS	weight	waist"	hips"
Beginning:	_____	_____	_____
End:	_____	_____	_____

233

NOVEMBER 4	BREAKFAST	LUNCH	DINNER	SNACKS
S M T W T F S Carbohydrate Total per Meal: B _____ L _____ D _____ S _____ Daily Carbohydrate Total: _____				
	Fluids: oz. Vit / Min / Supp:	Fluids: oz.	Fluids: oz.	Fluids: oz.

NOVEMBER 5	BREAKFAST	LUNCH	DINNER	SNACKS
S M T W T F S Carbohydrate Total per Meal: B _____ L _____ D _____ S _____ Daily Carbohydrate Total: _____				
	Fluids: oz. Vit / Min / Supp:	Fluids: oz.	Fluids: oz.	Fluids: oz.

NOVEMBER 6	BREAKFAST	LUNCH	DINNER	SNACKS
S M T W T F S Carbohydrate Total per Meal: B _____ L _____ D _____ S _____ Daily Carbohydrate Total: _____				
	Fluids: oz. Vit / Min / Supp:	Fluids: oz.	Fluids: oz.	Fluids: oz.

NOVEMBER 7	BREAKFAST	LUNCH	DINNER	SNACKS
S M T W T F S Carbohydrate Total per Meal: B _____ L _____ D _____ S _____ Daily Carbohydrate Total: _____				
	Fluids: oz. Vit / Min / Supp:	Fluids: oz.	Fluids: oz.	Fluids: oz.

EXERCISE GOALS: _____

EXERCISE DONE: _____

NOVEMBER 8	BREAKFAST	LUNCH	DINNER	SNACKS
S M T W T F S Carbohydrate Total per Meal: B _____ · L _____ D _____ S _____				
Daily Carbohydrate Total: _____	Fluids: _____ oz. Vit / Min / Supp:	Fluids: _____ oz.	Fluids: _____ oz.	Fluids: _____ oz.

NOVEMBER 9	BREAKFAST	LUNCH	DINNER	SNACKS
S M T W T F S Carbohydrate Total per Meal: B _____ L _____ D _____ S _____				
Daily Carbohydrate Total: _____	Fluids: _____ oz. Vit / Min / Supp:	Fluids: _____ oz.	Fluids: _____ oz.	Fluids: _____ oz.

NOVEMBER 10	BREAKFAST	LUNCH	DINNER	SNACKS
S M T W T F S Carbohydrate Total per Meal: B _____ L _____ D _____ S _____				
Daily Carbohydrate Total: _____	Fluids: _____ oz. Vit / Min / Supp:	Fluids: _____ oz.	Fluids: _____ oz.	Fluids: _____ oz.

TIP   Exercise. Exercise. Exercise. Begin where you are physically and set goals to increase your exercise as you progress. If you wish to join a gym, fine. However, you can walk without financial cost, and you can do calisthenics in your bedroom without cost. Check out a local church—they often have a free or very low cost exercise program. You might even catch a television exercise program.

QUOTE   "He who has health, has hope; and he who has hope, has everything." — Arabian proverb

GOAL FOR THE WEEK:

STATISTICS	weight	waist"	hips"
Beginning:	_____	_____	_____
End:	_____	_____	_____

NOVEMBER 11	BREAKFAST	LUNCH	DINNER	SNACKS
S M T W T F S Carbohydrate Total per Meal: B _____ L _____ D _____ S _____				•
Daily Carbohydrate Total: _____	Fluids: _____ oz.	Fluids: _____ oz.	Fluids: _____ oz.	Fluids: _____ oz.
	Vit / Min / Supp:			

NOVEMBER 12	BREAKFAST	LUNCH	DINNER	SNACKS
S M T W T F S Carbohydrate Total per Meal: B _____ L _____ D _____ S _____				
Daily Carbohydrate Total: _____	Fluids: _____ oz.	Fluids: _____ oz.	Fluids: _____ oz.	Fluids: _____ oz.
	Vit / Min / Supp:			

NOVEMBER 13	BREAKFAST	LUNCH	DINNER	SNACKS
S M T W T F S Carbohydrate Total per Meal: B _____ L _____ D _____ S _____				
Daily Carbohydrate Total: _____	Fluids: _____ oz.	Fluids: _____ oz.	Fluids: _____ oz.	Fluids: _____ oz.
	Vit / Min / Supp:			

NOVEMBER 14	BREAKFAST	LUNCH	DINNER	SNACKS
S M T W T F S Carbohydrate Total per Meal: B _____ L _____ D _____ S _____				
Daily Carbohydrate Total: _____	Fluids: _____ oz.	Fluids: _____ oz.	Fluids: _____ oz.	Fluids: _____ oz.
	Vit / Min / Supp:			

EXERCISE GOALS: _____

EXERCISE DONE: _____

NOVEMBER 15	BREAKFAST	LUNCH	DINNER	SNACKS
S M T W T F S Carbohydrate Total per Meal: B _____ L _____ D _____ S _____				
Daily Carbohydrate	Fluids: oz.	Fluids: oz.	Fluids: oz.	Fluids: oz.
Total: _____	Vit / Min / Supp:			

NOVEMBER 16	BREAKFAST	LUNCH	DINNER	SNACKS
S M T W T F S Carbohydrate Total per Meal: B _____ L _____ D _____ S _____				
Daily Carbohydrate	Fluids: oz.	Fluids: oz.	Fluids: oz.	Fluids: oz.
Total: _____	Vit / Min / Supp:			

NOVEMBER 17	BREAKFAST	LUNCH	DINNER	SNACKS
S M T W T F S Carbohydrate Total per Meal: B _____ L _____ D _____ S _____				
Daily Carbohydrate	Fluids: oz.	Fluids: oz.	Fluids: oz.	Fluids: oz.
Total: _____	Vit / Min / Supp:			

TIP   Turn on your favorite music and dance. Dance from the depths of your soul without a thought as to how it might look to anyone. Move as fully and freely as you can, truly expressing the music through your body. Doing this once a week for even ten minutes is healing for body and soul.

QUOTE   "When you get into a tight place and everything goes against you, till it seems as though you could not hold on a minute longer, never give up then, for that is just the place and time that the tide will turn."
— *Harriet Beecher Stowe*

GOAL FOR THE WEEK:

STATISTICS   weight   waist"   hips"
Beginning: _____   _____   _____
End: _____   _____   _____

NOVEMBER 18	BREAKFAST	LUNCH	DINNER	SNACKS
S M T W T F S Carbohydrate Total per Meal: B _____ L _____ D _____ S _____ Daily Carbohydrate Total: _____				
	Fluids: oz.	Fluids: oz.	Fluids: oz.	Fluids: oz.
	Vit / Min / Supp:			

NOVEMBER 19	BREAKFAST	LUNCH	DINNER	SNACKS
S M T W T F S Carbohydrate Total per Meal: B _____ L _____ D _____ S _____ Daily Carbohydrate Total: _____				
	Fluids: oz.	Fluids: oz.	Fluids: oz.	Fluids: oz.
	Vit / Min / Supp:			

NOVEMBER 20	BREAKFAST	LUNCH	DINNER	SNACKS
S M T W T F S Carbohydrate Total per Meal: B _____ L _____ D _____ S _____ Daily Carbohydrate Total: _____				
	Fluids: oz.	Fluids: oz.	Fluids: oz.	Fluids: oz.
	Vit / Min / Supp:			

NOVEMBER 21	BREAKFAST	LUNCH	DINNER	SNACKS
S M T W T F S Carbohydrate Total per Meal: B _____ L _____ D _____ S _____ Daily Carbohydrate Total: _____				
	Fluids: oz.	Fluids: oz.	Fluids: oz.	Fluids: oz.
	Vit / Min / Supp:			

EXERCISE GOALS: _____

EXERCISE DONE: _____

238

NOVEMBER 22	BREAKFAST	LUNCH	DINNER	SNACKS
S M T W T F S Carbohydrate Total per Meal: B _____ L _____ D _____ S _____ Daily Carbohydrate Total: _____				
	Fluids: _____ oz.	Fluids: _____ oz.	Fluids: _____ oz.	Fluids: _____ oz.
	Vit / Min / Supp:			

NOVEMBER 23	BREAKFAST	LUNCH	DINNER	SNACKS
S M T W T F S Carbohydrate Total per Meal: B _____ L _____ D _____ S _____ Daily Carbohydrate Total: _____				
	Fluids: _____ oz.	Fluids: _____ oz.	Fluids: _____ oz.	Fluids: _____ oz.
	Vit / Min / Supp:			

NOVEMBER 24	BREAKFAST	LUNCH	DINNER	SNACKS
S M T W T F S Carbohydrate Total per Meal: B _____ L _____ D _____ S _____ Daily Carbohydrate Total: _____				
	Fluids: _____ oz.	Fluids: _____ oz.	Fluids: _____ oz.	Fluids: _____ oz.
	Vit / Min / Supp:			

TIP Give thanks daily for all the things that are right in your life. Give thanks for all the progress you have made and all you will continue to make—every day.

QUOTE "Be not afraid of life. Believe that life is worth living, and your belief will help create the fact."
— William James

GOAL FOR THE WEEK:

STATISTICS	weight	waist"	hips"
Beginning:	_____	_____	_____
End:	_____	_____	_____

NOVEMBER 25	BREAKFAST	LUNCH	DINNER	SNACKS
S M T W T F S Carbohydrate Total per Meal: B _____ L _____ D _____ S _____				
Daily Carbohydrate	Fluids: _____ oz.	Fluids: _____ oz.	Fluids: _____ oz.	Fluids: _____ oz.
Total: _____	Vit / Min / Supp:			

NOVEMBER 26	BREAKFAST	LUNCH	DINNER	SNACKS
S M T W T F S Carbohydrate Total per Meal: B _____ L _____ D _____ S _____				
Daily Carbohydrate	Fluids: _____ oz.	Fluids: _____ oz.	Fluids: _____ oz.	Fluids: _____ oz.
Total: _____	Vit / Min / Supp:			

NOVEMBER 27	BREAKFAST	LUNCH	DINNER	SNACKS
S M T W T F S Carbohydrate Total per Meal: B _____ L _____ D _____ S _____				
Daily Carbohydrate	Fluids: _____ oz.	Fluids: _____ oz.	Fluids: _____ oz.	Fluids: _____ oz.
Total: _____	Vit / Min / Supp:			

NOVEMBER 28	BREAKFAST	LUNCH	DINNER	SNACKS
S M T W T F S Carbohydrate Total per Meal: B _____ L _____ D _____ S _____				
Daily Carbohydrate	Fluids: _____ oz.	Fluids: _____ oz.	Fluids: _____ oz.	Fluids: _____ oz.
Total: _____	Vit / Min / Supp:			

EXERCISE GOALS: _____

EXERCISE DONE: _____

NOVEMBER 29	BREAKFAST	LUNCH	DINNER	SNACKS
S M T W T F S Carbohydrate Total per Meal: B _____ L _____ D _____ S _____ Daily Carbohydrate Total: _____				
	Fluids: _____ oz.	Fluids: _____ oz.	Fluids: _____ oz.	Fluids: _____ oz.
	Vit / Min / Supp:			

NOVEMBER 30	BREAKFAST	LUNCH	DINNER	SNACKS
S M T W T F S Carbohydrate Total per Meal: B _____ L _____ D _____ S _____ Daily Carbohydrate Total: _____				
	Fluids: _____ oz.	Fluids: _____ oz.	Fluids: _____ oz.	Fluids: _____ oz.
	Vit / Min / Supp:			

DECEMBER 1	BREAKFAST	LUNCH	DINNER	SNACKS
S M T W T F S Carbohydrate Total per Meal: B _____ L _____ D _____ S _____ Daily Carbohydrate Total: _____				
	Fluids: _____ oz.	Fluids: _____ oz.	Fluids: _____ oz.	Fluids: _____ oz.
	Vit / Min / Supp:			

TIP   Don't bore yourself. If you've been exercising in the morning, change to evening. If you've been drinking tea, drink water. Take a shower instead of a bath, walk at a mall as opposed to your neighborhood—whatever it takes to keep you on the maintenance path.

QUOTE   "Man must be arched and buttressed from within, else the temple wavers to the dust." — *Marcus Aurelius*

GOAL FOR THE WEEK:

STATISTICS	weight	waist"	hips"
Beginning:	_____	_____	_____
End:	_____	_____	_____

DECEMBER 2	BREAKFAST	LUNCH	DINNER	SNACKS
S M T W T F S Carbohydrate Total per Meal: B _____ L _____ D _____ S _____				
Daily Carbohydrate Total: _____	Fluids: _____ oz.	Fluids: _____ oz.	Fluids: _____ oz.	Fluids: _____ oz.
	Vit / Min / Supp:			

DECEMBER 3	BREAKFAST	LUNCH	DINNER	SNACKS
S M T W T F S Carbohydrate Total per Meal: B _____ L _____ D _____ S _____				
Daily Carbohydrate Total: _____	Fluids: _____ oz.	Fluids: _____ oz.	Fluids: _____ oz.	Fluids: _____ oz.
	Vit / Min / Supp:			

DECEMBER 4	BREAKFAST	LUNCH	DINNER	SNACKS
S M T W T F S Carbohydrate Total per Meal: B _____ L _____ D _____ S _____				
Daily Carbohydrate Total: _____	Fluids: _____ oz.	Fluids: _____ oz.	Fluids: _____ oz.	Fluids: _____ oz.
	Vit / Min / Supp:			

DECEMBER 5	BREAKFAST	LUNCH	DINNER	SNACKS
S M T W T F S Carbohydrate Total per Meal: B _____ L _____ D _____ S _____				
Daily Carbohydrate Total: _____	Fluids: _____ oz.	Fluids: _____ oz.	Fluids: _____ oz.	Fluids: _____ oz.
	Vit / Min / Supp:			

EXERCISE GOALS: _____

EXERCISE DONE: _____

242

DECEMBER 6	BREAKFAST	LUNCH	DINNER	SNACKS
S M T W T F S Carbohydrate Total per Meal: B _____ L _____ D _____ S _____				
Daily Carbohydrate Total: _____	Fluids: _____ oz.	Fluids: _____ oz.	Fluids: _____ oz.	Fluids: _____ oz.
	Vit / Min / Supp:			

DECEMBER 7	BREAKFAST	LUNCH	DINNER	SNACKS
S M T W T F S Carbohydrate Total per Meal: B _____ L _____ D _____ S _____				
Daily Carbohydrate Total: _____	Fluids: _____ oz.	Fluids: _____ oz.	Fluids: _____ oz.	Fluids: _____ oz.
	Vit / Min / Supp:			

DECEMBER 8	BREAKFAST	LUNCH	DINNER	SNACKS
S M T W T F S Carbohydrate Total per Meal: B _____ L _____ D _____ S _____				
Daily Carbohydrate Total: _____	Fluids: _____ oz.	Fluids: _____ oz.	Fluids: _____ oz.	Fluids: _____ oz.
	Vit / Min / Supp:			

TIP   Broaden your palate. Foods you may never have liked before can offer new menu choices. Broccoli is good for you and very low in carbohydrates. Try it—you might like it, and you will surely like how much of it you can eat.

QUOTE   "Hope ever urges on and tells us tomorrow will be better." — *Albius Tibullus*

GOAL FOR THE WEEK:

STATISTICS	weight	waist"	hips"
Beginning:	_____	_____	_____
End:	_____	_____	_____

DECEMBER 9	BREAKFAST	LUNCH	DINNER	SNACKS
S M T W T F S Carbohydrate Total per Meal: B _____ L _____ D _____ S _____				
Daily Carbohydrate Total: _____	Fluids: oz.	Fluids: oz.	Fluids: oz.	Fluids: oz.
	Vit / Min / Supp:			

DECEMBER 10	BREAKFAST	LUNCH	DINNER	SNACKS
S M T W T F S Carbohydrate Total per Meal: B _____ L _____ D _____ S _____				
Daily Carbohydrate Total: _____	Fluids: oz.	Fluids: oz.	Fluids: oz.	Fluids: oz.
	Vit / Min / Supp:			

DECEMBER 11	BREAKFAST	LUNCH	DINNER	SNACKS
S M T W T F S Carbohydrate Total per Meal: B _____ L _____ D _____ S _____				
Daily Carbohydrate Total: _____	Fluids: oz.	Fluids: oz.	Fluids: oz.	Fluids: oz.
	Vit / Min / Supp:			

DECEMBER 12	BREAKFAST	LUNCH	DINNER	SNACKS
S M T W T F S Carbohydrate Total per Meal: B _____ L _____ D _____ S _____				
Daily Carbohydrate Total: _____	Fluids: oz.	Fluids: oz.	Fluids: oz.	Fluids: oz.
	Vit / Min / Supp:			

EXERCISE GOALS: _____

EXERCISE DONE: _____

DECEMBER 13	BREAKFAST	LUNCH	DINNER	SNACKS
S M T W T F S Carbohydrate Total per Meal: B _____ L _____ D _____ S _____				
Daily Carbohydrate Total: _____	Fluids: _____ oz.	Fluids: _____ oz.	Fluids: _____ oz.	Fluids: _____ oz.
	Vit / Min / Supp:			

DECEMBER 14	BREAKFAST	LUNCH	DINNER	SNACKS
S M T W T F S Carbohydrate Total per Meal: B _____ L _____ D _____ S _____				
Daily Carbohydrate Total: _____	Fluids: _____ oz.	Fluids: _____ oz.	Fluids: _____ oz.	Fluids: _____ oz.
	Vit / Min / Supp:			

DECEMBER 15	BREAKFAST	LUNCH	DINNER	SNACKS
S M T W T F S Carbohydrate Total per Meal: B _____ L _____ D _____ S _____				
Daily Carbohydrate Total: _____	Fluids: _____ oz.	Fluids: _____ oz.	Fluids: _____ oz.	Fluids: _____ oz.
	Vit / Min / Supp:			

TIP   Monitor that ongoing conversation you silently have with yourself—listen carefully. For every negative statement, mentally say, "Cancel that." Then reframe it to a positive affirmation. You'll be amazed at how many times you catch yourself putting yourself down.

QUOTE   "We are shaped and fashioned by what we love." — *Johann Wolfgang von Goethe*

GOAL FOR THE WEEK:

STATISTICS	weight	waist"	hips"
Beginning:	_____	_____	_____
End:	_____	_____	_____

DECEMBER 16	BREAKFAST	LUNCH	DINNER	SNACKS
S M T W T F S Carbohydrate Total per Meal: B _____ L _____ D _____ S _____ Daily Carbohydrate Total: _____				
	Fluids: oz.	Fluids: oz.	Fluids: oz.	Fluids: oz.
	Vit / Min / Supp:			

DECEMBER 17	BREAKFAST	LUNCH	DINNER	SNACKS
S M T W T F S Carbohydrate Total per Meal: B _____ L _____ D _____ S _____ Daily Carbohydrate Total: _____				
	Fluids: oz.	Fluids: oz.	Fluids: oz.	Fluids: oz.
	Vit / Min / Supp:			

DECEMBER 18	BREAKFAST	LUNCH	DINNER	SNACKS
S M T W T F S Carbohydrate Total per Meal: B _____ L _____ D _____ S _____ Daily Carbohydrate Total: _____				
	Fluids: oz.	Fluids: oz.	Fluids: oz.	Fluids: oz.
	Vit / Min / Supp:			

DECEMBER 19	BREAKFAST	LUNCH	DINNER	SNACKS
S M T W T F S Carbohydrate Total per Meal: B _____ L _____ D _____ S _____ Daily Carbohydrate Total: _____				
	Fluids: oz.	Fluids: oz.	Fluids: oz.	Fluids: oz.
	Vit / Min / Supp:			

EXERCISE GOALS: _____

EXERCISE DONE: _____

DECEMBER 20	BREAKFAST	LUNCH	DINNER	SNACKS
S M T W T F S Carbohydrate Total per Meal: B _____ L _____ D _____ S _____ Daily Carbohydrate Total: _____				
	Fluids: oz.	Fluids: oz.	Fluids: oz.	Fluids: oz.
	Vit / Min / Supp:			

DECEMBER 21	BREAKFAST	LUNCH	DINNER	SNACKS
S M T W T F S Carbohydrate Total per Meal: B _____ L _____ D _____ S _____ Daily Carbohydrate Total: _____				
	Fluids: oz.	Fluids: oz.	Fluids: oz.	Fluids: oz.
	Vit / Min / Supp:			

DECEMBER 22	BREAKFAST	LUNCH	DINNER	SNACKS
S M T W T F S Carbohydrate Total per Meal: B _____ L _____ D _____ S _____ Daily Carbohydrate Total: _____				
	Fluids: oz.	Fluids: oz.	Fluids: oz.	Fluids: oz.
	Vit / Min / Supp:			

TIP   If you can't decide whether or not to do something, ask yourself, "Will this action propel me toward my goals or keep me back?" Keeping on track with your goals is really being good to yourself.

QUOTE   "It is not true that love makes all things easy; it makes us choose what is difficult." — *George Eliot*

GOAL FOR THE WEEK:

STATISTICS	weight	waist"	hips"
Beginning:	_____	_____	_____
End:	_____	_____	_____

DECEMBER 23	BREAKFAST	LUNCH	DINNER	SNACKS
S M T W T F S Carbohydrate Total per Meal: B _____ L _____ D _____ S _____ Daily Carbohydrate Total: _____				
	Fluids: ___ oz.	Fluids: ___ oz.	Fluids: ___ oz.	Fluids: ___ oz.
	Vit / Min / Supp:			

DECEMBER 24	BREAKFAST	LUNCH	DINNER	SNACKS
S M T W T F S Carbohydrate Total per Meal: B _____ L _____ D _____ S _____ Daily Carbohydrate Total: _____				
	Fluids: ___ oz.	Fluids: ___ oz.	Fluids: ___ oz.	Fluids: ___ oz.
	Vit / Min / Supp:			

DECEMBER 25	BREAKFAST	LUNCH	DINNER	SNACKS
S M T W T F S Carbohydrate Total per Meal: B _____ L _____ D _____ S _____ Daily Carbohydrate Total: _____				
	Fluids: ___ oz.	Fluids: ___ oz.	Fluids: ___ oz.	Fluids: ___ oz.
	Vit / Min / Supp:			

DECEMBER 26	BREAKFAST	LUNCH	DINNER	SNACKS
S M T W T F S Carbohydrate Total per Meal: B _____ L _____ D _____ S _____ Daily Carbohydrate Total: _____				
	Fluids: ___ oz.	Fluids: ___ oz.	Fluids: ___ oz.	Fluids: ___ oz.
	Vit / Min / Supp:			

EXERCISE GOALS: _____

EXERCISE DONE: _____

DECEMBER 27	BREAKFAST	LUNCH	DINNER	SNACKS
S M T W T F S Carbohydrate Total per Meal: B _____ L _____ D _____ S _____				
Daily Carbohydrate Total: _____	Fluids: _____ oz.	Fluids: _____ oz.	Fluids: _____ oz.	Fluids: _____ oz.
	Vit / Min / Supp:			

DECEMBER 28	BREAKFAST	LUNCH	DINNER	SNACKS
S M T W T F S Carbohydrate Total per Meal: B _____ L _____ D _____ S _____				
Daily Carbohydrate Total: _____	Fluids: _____ oz.	Fluids: _____ oz.	Fluids: _____ oz.	Fluids: _____ oz.
	Vit / Min / Supp:			

DECEMBER 29	BREAKFAST	LUNCH	DINNER	SNACKS
S M T W T F S Carbohydrate Total per Meal: B _____ L _____ D _____ S _____				
Daily Carbohydrate Total: _____	Fluids: _____ oz.	Fluids: _____ oz.	Fluids: _____ oz.	Fluids: _____ oz.
	Vit / Min / Supp:			

TIP   Ponder the when, what, and why of your eating. When the urge to eat is upon you, stop and think. Try to figure out if you eat because you are angry, afraid, sad, lonesome, tired, or for any reason other than hunger. Then you can formulate a strategy to combat the real reason or at least be aware and override the urge.

QUOTE   "A loving heart is the truest wisdom." — *Charles Dickens*

GOAL FOR THE WEEK:

STATISTICS	weight	waist"	hips"
Beginning:	_____	_____	_____
End:	_____	_____	_____

DECEMBER 30	BREAKFAST	LUNCH	DINNER	SNACKS
S M T W T F S Carbohydrate Total per Meal: B _____ L _____ D _____ S _____ Daily Carbohydrate Total: _____				
	Fluids: oz.	Fluids: oz.	Fluids: oz.	Fluids: oz.
	Vit / Min / Supp:			

DECEMBER 31	BREAKFAST	LUNCH	DINNER	SNACKS
S M T W T F S Carbohydrate Total per Meal: B _____ L _____ D _____ S _____ Daily Carbohydrate Total: _____				
	Fluids: oz.	Fluids: oz.	Fluids: oz.	Fluids: oz.
	Vit / Min / Supp:			

QUOTES   "'How long does getting thin take?' Pooh asked anxiously." — *A. A. Milne*

"Looks can be deceiving—it's eating that's believing." — *James Thurber*

GOAL FOR THE WEEK:

STATISTICS	weight	waist"	hips"
Beginning:	_____	_____	_____
End:	_____	_____	_____

250

NOTES:

NOTES:

PROGRESS CHART

Week	WK 1	WK 2	WK 3	WK 4	WK 5	WK 6	WK 7	WK 8	WK 9	WK 10	WK 11	WK 12	WK 13	WK 14	WK 15	WK 16	WK 17	WK 18	WK 19	WK 20	WK 21	WK 22	WK 23	WK 23	WK 25	WK 26
Weight																										
Blood Pressure																										
Laboratory Tests																										
Total Cholesterol																										
HDL Cholesterol																										
LDL Cholesterol																										
Triglycerides																										
Triglyceride/ HDL																										
Glucose																										
Insulin																										
Other																										
Other																										
Other																										

PROGRESS CHART (continued)

Week	WK 27	WK 28	WK 29	WK 30	WK 31	WK 32	WK 33	WK 34	WK 35	WK 36	WK 37	WK 38	WK 39	WK 40	WK 41	WK 42	WK 43	WK 44	WK 45	WK 46	WK 46	WK 48	WK 49	WK 50	WK 51	WK 52
Weight																										
Blood Pressure																										
Laboratory Tests																										
Total Cholesterol																										
HDL Cholesterol																										
LDL Cholesterol																										
Triglycerides																										
Triglyceride/HDL																										
Glucose																										
Insulin																										
Other																										
Other																										
Other																										

Index

ACE inhibitors, 80
acid load. *See* bone loss
Agatson, Arthur, 78–79
alcohol, 56, 70–71, 79, 100
alpha lipoic acid, 113
anxiety, 63
arachidonic acid, 88, 105
artificial sweeteners, 111
aspartame, 111
assessment
    during maintenance, 36, 38–39,
      41–42, 44–45, 51–53
    during transition phase, 21, 31–34
    of weight, 51–52, 77–78, 82–83,
      110–112
athletes, 117–119. *See also* exercise
Atkins, Robert, 78
Atkins Diet, 78

bad breath, 104
beta-blockers, 80
beta shift, 107–108
beverages. *See* fluids
"Big 7" life stresses, 61–63. *See also*
    stress
bio-impedence technology, 82
blood pressure, 73–74, 76–77, 80
blood sugar
    glycemic index and, 79, 80–81
    glycerin and, 95

    Low-Carb Boot Camp and, 57
    See also diabetes; insulin
blood type, 79–80
bodybuilding, 118–119
body fat composition, 52
bone loss, 91–92, 121–122
breakfast, 69, 86–87, 93, 124
burger restaurants, 128
butter, 99

caffeine, 57
calcium channel blockers, 80
calories, 53–56
cancer, 122
canola oil, 98
Carbohydrate Addicts diet, 80
carbohydrates, 89–95
    "carb loading," 118
    Effective Carbohydrate Content
      (ECC), 78, 81, 90–91, 94
    intake balanced with output,
      53–56
    intake for maintenance, 7–9,
      35–37
    intake for transition phase, 11–14,
      32–34
    listing in Meal Planner Work-
      sheets, 18–20
    protein turned into, 85
    quality of, 14

carbohydrates (*continued*)
   sensitivity to, 13
   sources of, 89
cheese, 84, 99
chicken restaurants, 126–127
children, dieting by, 116–117
Chinese restaurants, 127
cholecystokinin (CCK), 96
cholesterol, 107–108
chromium polynicotinate, 113
clothing size, 52
coenzyme Q10, 113
coffee, 57
condiments, 100, 122–123
constipation, 104–105
control, 63–67
cooking methods, 88–89
coping strategies, 55
corrective phase, 49, 74–75
   meals for, 16–18
   setting goals for, 5–7
   See also weight loss
cottage cheese, 99
cravings, 124–125

D'Adamo, Peter, 79–80
daily journal, 4, 20, 109, 128–129
dairy, 84, 99
30-Day Low-Carb Diet Solution, The
   (Eades, Eades), 86, 93
depression, 63
desserts, 124
diabetes
   glycerin and, 95
   medication for, 73–74
   See also blood sugar; insulin
diarrhea, 95, 105
"dietary vacation," 49–50
diet goals, 1–4, 77–78

discipline and, 63–67
   interim, 5–7
   for transition phase, 11–14
discipline, 63–67
diuretics, 80
dizziness, 102
dressings, 57, 100, 123

Eades, Mary Dan and Michael R.
   Low-Carb Comfort Food Cook-
     book, The, 68, 69, 86, 87, 98,
     123
   Low-Carb CookwoRx (television
     program), 86, 99
   Protein Power, 13, 78, 82–83,
     86
   Protein Power LifePlan, The, 75,
     86
   Slow Burn Fitness Revolution,
     The, 119
   30-Day Low-Carb Diet Solution,
     The, 22
Eat Right for Your Blood Type diet,
   79–80
Effective Carbohydrate Content
   (ECC), 78, 81, 90–91, 94
eggs, 86–89
eicosanoids, 97
emotions, food and, 61–63
enzymes, 101
erythrotol, 94–95
estrogen replacement therapy,
   114–115
exercise, 119
   bodybuilding, 118–119
   carbohydrate intake and, 33–34,
     53
   muscle from, 110–112
   protein requirements and, 83

fast food restaurants, 126
fat
    ketone levels and, 102–104,
        108–109
    saturated, 79, 97
    sources of, 96–99
    transfats, 98
    weight measurement and, 51–52,
        77–78, 82–83, 110–112
fat calipers, 82
fiber, 78
fish oils, 96–97, 108
flaxseed oil, 96–97
fluids, 21–22
    importance of, 123
    during Low-Carb Boot Camp,
        57
    to reduce side effects, 102–103
    retention of, 52, 76–77
    weight loss and, 77–78, 81–82
food allergies, 98
food habits, 1–4, 50–51, 61–63
    binging, 49–50
    cravings, 124–125
    eating in restaurants, 126–128
    portion size and, 111
    traveling and, 125–126
food sensitivities, 87–89
food substitutions
    during holidays, 67–71
    during Low-Carb Boot Camp, 56
    stress and, 63
"free weekend plans," 49–50
fruits, 93–94

gastrointestinal (GI) discomfort, 95,
    104–105
Glasser, William, 66
glycemic index (GI), 79, 80–81

glycerin, 94, 95
glycogen, 118
goals. See diet goals
gout, 106
Gray, Charles, 118

Hahn, Fred, 119
hair loss, 105
Halloween, 67–68
hamburger restaurants, 128
HDL, 107–108
headaches, 102–103
health issues, 114–120
    food sensitivities and, 87–88
    medication for, 73–74
    monitoring, 52
    myths about low-carb dieting and,
        120–122
Heller, Rachel, 80
Heller, Richard, 80
holidays, diet during, 67–71
hormones
    fluid retention and, 52
    replacement therapy, 114–115
hydrostatic body fat test, 82
hypokalemia, 103

insulin, 74–75
    artificial sweeteners and, 111
    carbohydrate intake and, 91–93
    estrogen and, 114–115
    glycerin and, 95
    Low-Carb Boot Camp and, 57
    medication levels and, 73–74
    morning sensitivity to, 69, 86–87,
        93, 124
    resistance, 53
    uric acid and, 106
    See also blood sugar; diabetes

iron, 112
Italian restaurants, 127

Japanese restaurants, 127–128
journals, food, 4, 20, 109, 128–129

ketone levels, 102–104, 108–109
kidneys, 84, 107, 113–120, 120–121

labels. *See* nutrition labels
lactation, 115–116
lactitol, 94–95
LDL, 107–108
leftover food, 69
lightheadedness, 102
Low-Carb Boot Camp, 50, 56–61,
    112
Low-Carb Comfort Food Cookbook,
    The (Eades, Eades), 68, 69, 86,
    87, 98, 123, 124–125
Low-Carb CookwoRx (television
    program), 86, 99
low-carb diets
    comparison of, 78–80
    foods to avoid, 122–123
    myths about, 120–122
    Protein Power, described, 74–76.
        See also individual book names
    side effects of, 101–109

macadamia nuts, 100
magnesium, 57, 76–77, 101, 102, 112
maintenance, 1–4, 35–37, 74–76,
    119–120
    apprehension about, 7–9
    assessment during, 36, 38–39,
        41–42, 44–45, 51–53
    balancing strategies for, 49–51,
        53–56

benefits of, 9–10
discipline and, 63–67
during holidays, 67–71
mind-set for, 71–72
readiness for, 5–7
maltitol, 94–95
mayonnaise, 98–99
Meal Planner Worksheet, 18–20
meal plans, 14–16
    for corrective phase, 16–18
    for Low-Carb Boot Camp, 57–61
    for transition phase, 14–18, 22–31
meat
    alternatives to, 22, 85–86, 117
    avoidance of, 87–88
    quantity of, 88–89
    uric acid levels and, 106
medication, 73–74, 80
menopause, 115
menstruation, 114–115
metabolism, 14, 33, 35
    binging and, 50
    eliminating carbohydrates and, 92
milk, 99
muscle, increase of, 110–112
muscle cramps, 103

nails, 106
Naval Health Research Center, 118
"net Atkins carb count," 78
nursing mothers, 115–116
nutrition labels, 90–91, 93–95
nuts, 97–98, 100

omega-3 oils, 96–97
osteoporosis, 91–92, 121–122

parties, eating at, 70–71
pattern A/B cholesterol, 107–108

peanuts, 98
pentabosol, 114
physical activity. *See* exercise
Physician's Information Packet, 74
pizza restaurants, 127
plateau, weight loss, 109–112
pork chop restaurants, 126–127
potassium, 57, 76–77, 101–103,
    112–113
pregnancy, 6, 115–116
Progress Chart, 6, 34, 129
protein
    body's use of, 84–86
    lean body mass assessment,
        82–83
    listing in Meal Planner Work-
        sheets, 18–20
    myths about low-carb dieting and,
        120–122
    requirements, 15, 82, 115–117
    sources of, 83–84, 86–89
Protein Power Bulletin Board,
    73
Protein Power diet
    compared to other low-carb diets,
        78–80
    description of, 74–76
    See also individual book names
Protein Power (Eades, Eades), 13,
    78, 82–83, 86
Protein Power LifePlan, The (Eades,
    Eades), 75, 86, 112

restaurants, ordering in, 126–128

saturated fats, 79, 97
seafood restaurants, 126–127
Sears, Barry, 79
self-control, 63–67

7-Day Low-Carb Boot Camp, 50,
    56–61, 112
shellfish, uric acid levels and, 106
sleep, 103–104
Slow Burn Fitness Revolution, The
    (Eades, Eades, Hahn), 119
snacking, 123
    during Low-Carb Boot Camp,
        56
    during transition phase, 20–21
sodium, 102
sorbitol, 94–95
soup, 69
South Beach Diet, 78–79, 96, 100
steak restaurants, 126–127
stress, 55, 61–63
submarine sandwich restaurants, 127
sugar alcohols, 94–95
Sugar Busters diet, 79
supplements, 57
    for cholesterol, 108
    magnesium, 57, 76–77, 101, 102,
        112
    potassium, 57, 76–77, 101, 102,
        112
    recommendations, 112–114
    for side effects, 101–103, 106

Take Effective Control of Your Life
    (Glasser), 66
Tanita method, of lean body mass
    calculation, 82
Thai restaurants, 127
30-Day Low-Carb Diet Solution, The
    (Eades, Eades), 22
365-day Staying Power LifePlanner
    journal, 4, 20, 109, 128–129
tiredness, 101
transfats, 98

transition phase, 74–76
  assessment, 21, 31–34
  length of, 21
  meal plans for, 14–18, 22–31
  setting goals for, 11–14
  snacks for, 20–21
traveling, diet tips for, 125–126
triglycerides, 107–108

vegetables, 93–94
vegetarianism, 22, 117, 122. See *also*
    protein
Vietnamese restaurants, 127
vitamin A, 106
vitamin E, 113–114
vitamins. *See* supplements; *individual*
    vitamin names
vitamin supplements. *See* supple-
    ments

water. *See* fluids
weakness, 101

weight loss
  during corrective phase, 5–7,
      16–18, 49, 74–75, 93
  eliminating carbohydrates and,
      91–92
  goals for, 1–4, 11–14, 63–67,
      77–78
  plateau, 109–112
weight measurement, 51–52, 77–78,
    82–83, 110–112
Willet, Walter, 78, 79
women
  dieting while pregnant/lactating, 6,
      115–116
  hormonal changes in, 114–115
  weight fluctuation in, 52

xylitol, 94–95

yogurt, 99

Zone diet, 79, 96

Also by Drs. Michael and Mary Dan Eades

The following books are available at bookstores nationwide and online:

Protein Power (Bantam Books, 1996)

The Protein Power LifePlan (Warner Books, 2000)

The Protein Power LifePlan Gram Counter (Warner Books, 2000)

The Slow Burn Fitness Revolution (Broadway, 2003)

The 30-Day Low-Carb Diet Solution (Wiley, 2003)

The Low-Carb Comfort Food Cookbook (Wiley, 2003)

Beginning in April 2005, tune in each week to catch the Drs. Eades in the kitchen on their new PBS cooking series, *Low-Carb CookwoRx*. To find out more, visit us online at www.lowcarbcookworx.com.

For supplement information, related sources, recommended reading, health and nutrition tips, an online body-fat calculator, low-carbers' bulletin board and support groups, and more, visit us online at the official Drs. Eades Web site, www.proteinpower.com.

For more information about the Pentabosol weight loss supplement, visit www.pentabosol.com.